O D L

OXFORD DIABETES LIBRARY

Heart Disease and Diabetes

O D L

OXFORD DIABETES LIBRARY

Heart Disease and Diabetes

SECOND EDITION

Edited by

Professor Miles Fisher

Consultant Physician,
Glasgow Royal Infirmary,
UK

OXFORD
UNIVERSITY PRESS

OXFORD
UNIVERSITY PRESS

Great Clarendon Street, Oxford OX2 6DP,
United Kingdom

Oxford University Press is a department of the University of Oxford.
It furthers the University's objective of excellence in research, scholarship,
and education by publishing worldwide. Oxford is a registered trade mark of
Oxford University Press in the UK and in certain other countries

© Oxford University Press 2012

The moral rights of the authors have been asserted

First Edition published 2009
Second Edition published 2012

Impression: 1

British Library Cataloguing in Publication Data

Data available

Library of Congress Cataloging in Publication Data

Data available

ISBN 978-0-19-960456-2

Printed in Great Britain by
Clays Ltd, St Ives plc

Oxford University Press makes no representation, express or implied, that the
drug dosages in this book are correct. Readers must therefore always check
the product information and clinical procedures with the most up-to-date
published product information and data sheets provided by the manufacturers
and the most recent codes of conduct and safety regulations. The authors and
the publishers do not accept responsibility or legal liability for any errors in the
text or for the misuse or misapplication of material in this work. Except where
otherwise stated, drug dosages and recommendations are for the non-pregnant
adult who is not breast-feeding.

Links to third party websites are provided by Oxford in good faith and for
information only. Oxford disclaims any responsibility for the materials contained
in any third party website referenced in this work.

Contents

Preface

The management of people with type 1 and type 2 diabetes has improved following the results of large multi-centre trials. The microvascular complications of retinopathy, nephropathy, and neuropathy can all be reduced by intensive glycaemic control. Long-term epidemiological follow-up from trials has now shown that intensive glycaemic control reduces macrovascular complications, especially coronary events.

The focus has therefore shifted from whether improved glycaemic control reduces cardiovascular events, to identifying the safest treatment regimen for improving glycaemic control without unacceptable weight gain or hypoglycaemia.

Further advances have also been made in the management of dyslipidaemia and hypertension in diabetes, and there have been several well designed and well-conducted studies examining the most appropriate cardiovascular intervention for diabetic patients with established coronary heart disease.

This second edition of the book remains a concise and practical guide to reducing cardiovascular risk and in particular heart disease in people with diabetes. It will be of interest to GPs and practice nurses, hospital specialists, and specialist nurses in diabetes and cardiology, and has been extensively up-dated to reflect the results of recent trials.

As for the first edition I am extremely grateful to the other authors for their contributions to this book. Stephen Wheatcroft and his cardiology colleagues from Leeds have provided the more cardiological chapters, and Chapter 7 on coronary revascularization in the patient with diabetes has been heavily revised. Again my diabetes work colleague Ken Paterson, along with clinical pharmacology colleagues has produced a very useful and understandable guide to the heath economic aspects of treating cardiovascular disease in diabetes.

In producing this second edition my wife Margaret and son Marc have caught me sneaking off to work on the laptop at weekends and evenings, and I thank them for their continuing support and patience.

Miles Fisher, December 2010

Abbreviations

ABPM	Ambulatory blood pressure monitoring
ACE	Angiotensin-converting enzyme
ACS	Acute coronary syndrome
ADVANCE	Action in Diabetes and Vascular disease: preterAx and diamicroN-MR Controlled Evaluation
ACCOMPLISH	Avoiding Cardiovascular Events through Combination Therapy in Patients Living with Systolic Hypertension
ACCORD	Action to Control Cardiovascular Risk in Diabetes
AGE	Advanced glycation end products
ALLHAT	Antihypertensive and Lipid-Lowering treatment to prevent Heart Attack Trial
ARA	Angiotensin-II receptor antagonists
ARTS	Arterial Revascularization Therapies Study
ASCOT	Anglo-Scandinavian Cardiac Outcomes Trial
ATP	Adult Treatment Panel
AWESOME	Angina With Extremely Serious Operative Mortality Evaluation
BARI	Bypass Angioplasty Revascularization
BARI 2-D	Bypass Angioplasty Revascularization Investigation 2 Diabetes
BNP	Brain natriuretic peptide
CABG	Coronary artery bypass graft
CABRI	Coronary Angioplasty versus Bypass Revascularization Investigation
CANOE	Canadian Normoglycaemia Outcomes Evaluation
CAPRIE	Clopidogrel versus Aspirin in Patients at Risk of Ischemic Events
CARDS	Collaborative AtoRvastatin Diabetes Study
CARE	Cholesterol and Recurrent Events
CHD	Coronary heart disease

CHF	Chronic heart failure
CIMT	Carotid intima-media thickness
CKD	Chronic kidney disease
CORE	Centre for Outcomes Research
COURAGE	Clinical Outcomes Utilizing Revascularization and Aggressive Drug Evaluation
CRP	C-reactive protein
CTT	Cholesterol Treatment Trialists
CURE	Clopidogrel in Unstable Angina to Prevent Recurrent Events'
CVD	Cerebrovascular disease
DCCT	Diabetes Control and Complications Trial
DETAIL	Diabetics Exposed to Telmisartan and Enalapril
DIABHYCAR	Diabetes, Hypertension, cardiovascular events, and Ramipril
DIAD	Detection of Silent Myocardial Ischaemic in Asymptomatic Diabetics
DIGAMI	Diabetes Mellitus Insulin Glucose Infusion in Acute Myocardial Infarction
DiGEM	Diabetes glycaemic education and monitoring
DPP	Diabetes Prevention Program
DPS	Diabetes Prevention Study
DREAM	Diabetes Reduction Assessment with ramipril and rosiglitazone Medication
EAST	Emory Angioplasty versus Surgery Trial
EBCT	Electron-beam computed tomography
ECG	Electrocardiography
ED	Erectile dysfunction
EDIC	Epidemiology of Diabetes Interventions and Complications
ESRD	End-stage renal disease
EUROPA	EURopean trial On reduction of cardiac events with Perindopril in stable coronary Artery disease
FDA	Federal Drug Administration
GIP	Glucose-dependent insulinotropic peptide
GIST-UK	UK Glucose Insulin in Stroke Trial
GRACE	Global Registry of Acute Coronary Events
HDL	High-density lipoprotein

HDS	Hypertension in Diabetes Study
HI-5	Hyperglycemia Intensive Insulin Infusion in Infarction
HOPE	Heart Outcomes Prevention Evaluation
HOT	Hypertension Optimal Treatment trial
HPS	Heart Protection Study
HR	Hazard ratios
HYVET	Hypertension in the Very Elderly Trial
ICD	Implantable cardiac defibrillators
ICER	Incremental cost-effectiveness ratio
IDNT	Irbesartan Diabetic Nephropathy Trial
IFG	Impaired fasting glucose
IGT	Impaired glucose tolerance
IRMA-2	Irbesartan in Patients with Type 2 Diabetes and Microalbuminuria Study
JBS 2	Joint British Societies' Guidelines on prevention of cardiovascular disease in clinical practice
JUPITER	Justification for the Use of statins in Prevention: an Intervention Trial Evaluating Rosuvastatin
LAGB	Laparoscopic adjustable gastric banding
LDL	Low-density lipoprotein
LIFE	Losartan Intervention For Endpoint reduction in hypertension
LIPID	Long-Term Intervention with Pravastatin in Ischaemic Disease
LMWH	Low molecular weight heparins
LVSD	Left ventricular systolic dysfunction
MARVAL	Microalbuminuria Reduction with Valsartan
MI	Myocardial infarction
MIBG	Meta-iodobenzylguanidine
MICRO-HOPE	Microalbuminuria, Cardiovascular and Renal Outcomes-Heart Outcomes Prevention Evaluation
MRI	Magnetic resonance imaging
MSCT	Multi-slice computed tomography
NAVIGATOR	Nateglinide and Valsartan in Impaired Glucose Tolerance Outcomes Research
NICE	National Institute for Health and Clinical Excellence

NO	Nitric oxide
NOD	New-onset diabetes
NYHA	New York Heart Association
OGTT	Oral glucose tolerance test
PAD	Peripheral arterial disease
PCI	Percutaneous coronary intervention
PCI-CURE	Clopidogrel in Unstable angina to Reduce Recurrent Events (CURE) trial of patients with acute coronary syndromes undergoing PCI
PEACE	Prevention of Events with Angiotensin Converting Enzyme inhibition
PPAR	Peroxisome proliferator-activated receptor
PROactive	PROspective pioglitAzone Clinical Trial In macroVascular Events
PROGRESS	Perindopril Protection against Recurrent Stroke Study
PROVE-IT TIMI 22	Pravastatin or Atorvastatin Evaluation and Infection Therapy-Thrombolysis in Myocardial Infraction 22
PTCA	Percutaneous Transluminal Coronary Angioplasty
QALY	Quality adjusted life year
RCT	Randomized controlled trial
REACH	Reduction of Atherthrombosis for Continued Health
RECORD	Rosiglitazone Evaluated for Cardiac Outcomes and Regulation of glycaemia in Diabetes
RENAAL	Reduction of Endpoints in NIDDM with the Angiotensin II Antagonist Losartan
SCOUT	Sibutramine Cardiovascular Outcomes Trial
SHEP	Systolic Hypertension in the Elderly Program
SMC	Scottish Medicines Consortium
SOS	Stents or Surgery
SPARCL	Stroke Prevention by Aggressive Reduction in Cholesterol Levels
SPECT	Single-photon emission computed tomography
STOP-NIDDM	Study to Prevent Non-Insulin-Dependent Diabetes Mellitus
SYNTAX	SYNergy between percutaneous coronary intervention with TAXus and cardiac surgery

TIA	Transient ischaemic attacks
TNT	Treatment to New Targets
TREAT	Trial to Reduce Cardiovascular Events with Aranesp Therapy
TRITON-TIMI 38	Trial to Assess Improvement in Therapeutic Outcomes by Optimizing Platelet Inhibition with Prasugrel-Thrombolysis in Myocardial Infarction 38
TZD	Thiazolidinedione
UFH	Unfractionated heparin
UKPDS	United Kingdom Prospective Diabetes Study
VLDL	Very low-density lipoprotein
WHO	World Health Organization
WOSCOPS	West of Scotland Coronary Prevention Study
XENDOS	XENical in the prevention of Diabetes in Obese Subjects

Contributors

Dr Owen Bebb

Clinical Research Fellow,
Division of Cardiovascular &
Diabetes Research,
Leeds Institute of Genetics,
Health and Therapeutics,
LIGHT Laboratories
University of Leeds,
Leeds, UK

Ms Ailsa Brown

Principal Health Economist,
Scottish Medicines Consortium,
Glasgow, UK

Ms Joyce Craig

Lead Health Economist,
NHS Quality Improvement,
Glasgow, UK

Professor Miles Fisher

Consultant Physician,
Glasgow Royal Infirmary,
Glasgow, UK

Dr Matthew Kahn BSc, MRCP

Clinical Research Fellow,
Division of Cardiovascular and .
Diabetes Research,
Leeds Institute of Genetics,
Health & Therapeutics
LIGHT Laboratories,
University of Leeds,
Leeds, UK

Professor Ken Paterson

Consultant Physician,
Glasgow Royal Infirmary,
Glasgow, UK

Dr Adil Rajwani BSc, MRCP

Clinical Research Fellow,
Division of Cardiovascular and
Diabetes Research,
Leeds Institute of Genetics,
Health & Therapeutics
LIGHT Laboratories,
University of Leeds,
Leeds, UK

Dr Stephen Wheatcroft BSc, PhD, MRCP

British Heart Foundation
Intermediate Clinical Research
Fellow/Consultant Cardiologist
Division of Cardiovascular and
Diabetes Research,
Leeds Institute of Genetics,
Health & Therapeutics
LIGHT Laboratories,
University of Leeds,
Leeds, UK

Chapter 1

Introduction, epidemiology, and cardiovascular risk factors

Miles Fisher

Diabetes is a state of premature cardiovascular death which is associated with chronic hyperglycaemia and may also be associated with blindness and renal failure

Miles Fisher, British Diabetic Association meeting Dublin 1996.

Key points

- Cardiovascular disease is a common cause of morbidity and mortality in people with type 2 diabetes. Some guidelines define diabetes as a coronary heart disease equivalent, requiring multiple cardiovascular risk factor reduction
- In addition to diabetes the WHO has defined impaired glucose tolerance and impaired fasting glucose as intermediate hyperglycaemia. Subjects with intermediate hyperglycaemia have an increased risk of cardiovascular disease, and of progression to diabetes
- The presence of the metabolic syndrome (abdominal obesity, diabetes or impaired fasting glucose, raised blood pressure, and dyslipidaemia) predicts subsequent development of diabetes and vascular disease, but is not a separate target for intervention
- The relative risk of cardiovascular disease is greatly increased in people with type 1 diabetes, but the absolute risk is not particularly high. Components of the metabolic syndrome predict cardiovascular risk in type 1 diabetes.

1.1 Introduction

When I suggested the above re-definition of diabetes, which was prior to the publication of the results of the United Kingdom Prospective Diabetes Study (UKPDS), only the treatment of hyper-cholesterolaemia and hypertension, plus the use of antiplatelet drugs in certain high-risk patients, were of proven benefit in reducing cardiovascular events in people with diabetes. The purpose of the re-definition was to awaken healthcare professionals caring for people with diabetes to the fact that clinical management needed to embrace the prevention, detection and treatment of macrovascular disease in addition to microvascular disease.

1.2 Epidemiology

The Framingham study was one of the first to quantify the increased risk of cardiovascular morbidity and mortality in people with diabetes, and showed that there was an excess of cardiovascular disease in people with diabetes (predominantly type 2 diabetes) compared to non-diabetic people. This could not be fully explained by conventional cardiovascular risk factors of blood pressure, cholesterol, smoking, or obesity. Excesses were demonstrated in coronary heart disease, congestive cardiac failure, strokes, peripheral vascular disease and cardiovascular deaths (Table 1.1). In particular, an excess cardiovascular morbidity and mortality was seen in women with diabetes, and the rates of vascular disease in diabetic women approached the rates of vascular disease in men with diabetes.

In a population-based study from Finland it was shown that people with type 2 diabetes, who had no known cardiac disease, had the same incidence of myocardial infarction and cardiovascular death on 7-year follow-up as people without diabetes who had sustained

Table 1.1 Increased risk of cardiovascular disease in diabetic subjects compared to non-diabetic subjects in the Framingham study		
	Relative risk men	Relative risk women
Coronary heart disease	2	3
Stroke	2	4
Peripheral arterial disease	4	6
Congestive heart failure	2	5
Any cardiovascular disease	2	3
Cardiovascular death	2	5

Figure 1.1 Hazard ratios (HRs) for vascular outcomes in people with diabetes at baseline versus those without diabetes from the Emerging Risk Factors Collaboration

	Number of cases	HR (95% CI)	I^2 (95% CI)
Coronary heart disease*	26505	2.00 (1.83–2.19)	64 (54–71)
Coronary death	11556	2.31 (2.05–2.60)	41 (24–54)
Non-fatal myocardial infarction	14741	1.82 (1.64–2.03)	37 (19–51)
Stroke subtypes*			
Ischaemic stroke	3799	2.27 (1.95–2.65)	1 (0–20)
Haemorrhagic stroke	1183	1.56 (1.19–2.05)	0 (0–26)
Unclassified stroke	4973	1.84 (1.59–2.13)	33 (12–48)
Other vascular deaths	3826	1.73 (1.51–1.90)	0 (0–26)

Reprinted from *The Lancet*, **375**, The Emerging Risk Factors Collaboration. Diabetes mellitus, fasting blood glucose concentration, and risk of vascular disease: a collaborative meta-analysis of 102 prospective studies, 2215–2222. Copyright (2010), with permission from Elsevier.

a myocardial infarction. Similar results were obtained on 18-year follow-up. Others later challenged the suggestion that diabetes is a true coronary heart disease equivalent, pointing out that while the event rate in people with diabetes who are completely free of vascular disease at baseline is increased compared to non-diabetic subjects, the event rate is not as high as in survivors of myocardial infarction.

A recent meta-analysis from the Emerging Risk Factors Collaboration has been performed of 102 prospective studies containing 698,782 people without initial vascular disease. Risks for coronary heart disease were doubled in people with diabetes (Figure 1.1), and for women with diabetes the risk was greatest.

1.2.1 Risk factors for coronary heart disease in diabetes

The UKPDS was a large randomized trial of intensive versus conventional treatment of blood glucose in recently diagnosed patients with type 2 diabetes. A large amount of epidemiological data has been obtained from the study. In the UKPDS at baseline the traditional risk markers of hypertension, dyslipidaemia, and smoking, as well as HbA1c were independent risk factors for subsequent coronary events, indicating a potential for risk factor intervention in people with type 2 diabetes (Table 1.2). The importance of HbA1c as a risk factor is that it indicated that it was not just the presence of diabetes but the degree of hyperglycaemia as measured by HbA1c that was important. Variation in fasting blood glucose and HbA1c within the normal range has been shown to predict cardiovascular risk within

Table 1.2 Risk factors for coronary heart disease and myocardial infarction in the UKPDS (UKPDS 23, Turner et al., 1998)

Coronary artery disease	Fatal or non-fatal myocardial infarction	Fatal myocardial infarction
Raised LDL cholesterol	Raised LDL cholesterol	Diastolic blood pressure
Low HDL cholesterol	Diastolic blood pressure	Raised LDL cholesterol
HbA1c	Smoking	HbA1c
Systolic blood pressure	Low HDL cholesterol	
Smoking	HbA1c	

Reproduced from Turner RC, Millins H, Neil HAW, Stratton IM, Manley SE, Matthews DR, Holman RR (1998) Risk factors for coronary artery disease in non-insulin dependent diabetes mellitus: United Kingdom Prospective Diabetes Study (UKPDS: 23). *British Medical Journal*: **316**: 823–8, with permission from BMJ Publishing Group Ltd.

the non-diabetic population. In this way, glycaemia as a risk factor is similar to cholesterol and blood pressure (Figure 1.2).

More recently several novel risk markers have been shown to predict cardiovascular risk in diabetes, including endothelial dysfunction, microalbuminuria and reduced estimated glomerular filtration rate, fibrinogen and other markers of haemostasis, and C-reactive protein (CRP) and other markers of inflammation.

Figure 1.2 Comparison of hazard ratios (HRs) for coronary heart disease by long-term average concentrations of fasting blood glucose, total (and non-HDL) cholesterol and systolic blood pressure, from the Emerging Risk Factors Collaboration

Reprinted from *The Lancet*, **375**, The Emerging Risk Factors Collaboration. Diabetes mellitus, fasting blood glucose concentration, and risk of vascular disease: a collaborative meta-analysis of 102 prospective studies, 2215–2222. Copyright (2010), with permission from Elsevier.

1.2.2 Risk estimation

Cardiovascular risk tables have been used to estimate risk in asymptomatic individuals, and to make decisions on possible treatment of dyslipidaemia or hypertension. Many risk tables are based on data obtained from Framingham. This method of risk estimation is much less accurate in diabetic subjects for several reasons:

- There were few subjects with diabetes in the Framingham cohort that was used to derive the Framingham equation.
- The typical dyslipidaemia of diabetes comprises a relatively normal total cholesterol or LDL cholesterol, but with a higher concentration of the more atherogenic small dense LDL (Chapter 3).
- Patients were not characterized according to type of diabetes, and most were presumed to have type 2 diabetes in this age group, so data are lacking for patients with type 1 diabetes.
- Framingham studied a largely white population, so does not take account of ethnicity. It has been shown that many diabetic ethnic minority groups, such as South Asians in the UK, are at a higher cardiovascular risk than the majority population.
- It does not take account of microalbuminuria or novel risk markers.

A possible solution to this problem is to use a method of estimating risk that is unique for diabetes, such as the UKPDS risk engine. Another approach is to accept that people with diabetes have a coronary risk equivalent to existing coronary heart disease in non-diabetic subjects and to treat accordingly. This approach was first adopted in the Adult Treatment Panel (ATP) III guidelines in the US, and in the UK by the revised Joint British Societies' Guidelines on prevention of cardiovascular disease in clinical practice (JBS 2).

1.3 Intermediate hyperglycaemia

The WHO diagnostic criteria for the diagnosis of diabetes are based on the subsequent development of microvascular complications, particularly retinopathy, and not macrovascular complications. Two categories of intermediate hyperglycaemia, sometimes called 'pre-diabetes', are also described-impaired glucose tolerance and impaired fasting glucose (Table 1.3). Both of these predict the subsequent development of diabetes, and are associated with an increased risk of cardiovascular disease. Impaired glucose tolerance (IGT) is a better predictor of cardiovascular disease than impaired fasting glucose (IFG), supporting the suggesting that post-prandial glucose excursions may be a more important contributor to vascular events than fasting glucose. A raised HbA1c of 6.5% or above was recently added to the diagnostic criteria for diabetes.

Table 1.3 Diagnostic criteria for diabetes, impaired glucose tolerance, and impaired fasting glucose

Diabetes mellitus	Impaired glucose tolerance	Impaired fasting glucose
Random plasma glucose ≥ 11.1 mmol/L *Or* Fasting plasma glucose ≥ 7.0 mmol/L *Or* 2 hour plasma glucose ≥ 11.1 mmol/L on oral glucose tolerance test (OGTT)	Fasting plasma glucose < 7.0 mmol/L *And* 2 hour plasma glucose 7.8–11.0 mmol/L on OGTT	Fasting plasma glucose 6.0–6.9 mmol/lL (WHO criteria) *Or* Fasting plasma glucose 5.6–6.9 (ADA criteria)

The progression from intermediate hyperglycaemia to diabetes can be delayed by changes in lifestyle and pharmacological therapy, but so far only acarbose has been shown to reduce cardiovascular events (Table 1.4).

1.3.1 Lifestyle measures in intermediate hyperglycaemia

The effects of changes in diet and increased physical activity on the progression to diabetes were examined in the Finnish Diabetes Prevention Study (DPS) and the Diabetes Prevention Program (DPP) from the US. In the DPP, lifestyle change was more effective than metformin in reducing the progression to diabetes. Changes in cardiovascular risk factors are shown in Table 1.4. Observational follow-up of the DPP is being performed to see if these changes in cardiovascular risk factors lead to a reduction in cardiovascular events.

Table 1.4 Effects of interventions to reduce the progression to diabetes on cardiovascular risk markers or cardiovascular events

Intervention	Effect on cardiovascular risk
Lifestyle change	Reduced weight, blood pressure, triglycerides, increased HDL cholesterol, improved fibrinolysis
Metformin	Reduced weight
Acarbose	Reduced major cardiovascular events and new hypertension
Orlistat	Reduced blood pressure, total and LDL cholesterol
Rosiglitazone	Increased weight, insignificant increase in cardiovascular events
Pioglitazone	Increased weight, reduced triglycerides, reduced diastolic blood pressure, increased HDL cholesterol
Nateglinide	No beneficial effect

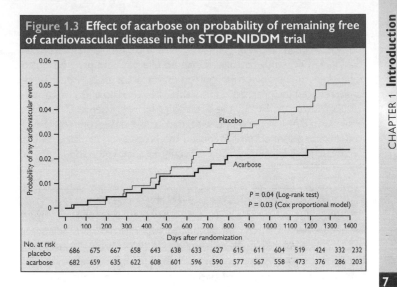

Figure 1.3 Effect of acarbose on probability of remaining free of cardiovascular disease in the STOP-NIDDM trial

1.3.2 Acarbose in intermediate hyperglycaemia

In the Study to Prevent Non-Insulin-Dependent Diabetes Mellitus (STOP-NIDDM) trial acarbose delayed the progression to diabetes in patients with IGT. Similar results were obtained with voglibose in a study from Japan. In a post-hoc analysis from STOP-NIDDM patients in the acarbose group had a significant reduction in a cardiovascular composite outcome that included coronary heart disease, cardiovascular death, congestive cardiac failure, strokes, and peripheral vascular disease (Figure 1.3). There was also a significant reduction in the development of hypertension.

1.3.3 Orlistat in intermediate hyperglycaemia

In the XENical in the prevention of Diabetes in Obese Subjects (XENDOS) study orlistat delayed the progression to diabetes, particularly in subjects with IGT. Weight was reduced with orlistat, and there were greater reductions in systolic and diastolic blood pressure, total and LDL cholesterol. HbA1c and cardiovascular events were not reported.

1.3.4 Other drugs in intermediate hyperglycaemia

One arm of the DPP was the use of troglitazone, but this arm was discontinued because of hepatic toxicity, including a subject in DPP who died from liver failure. In the Diabetes Reduction Assessment with ramipril and rosiglitazone Medication (DREAM) study rosiglitazone was highly effective at reducing the progression to diabetes, but a non-significant increase in cardiovascular events was observed (see also Chapter 2). In the smaller Actos Now for the Prevention of Diabetes (ACT NOW) study pioglitazone reduced the progression to diabetes and had beneficial effects on several cardiovascular risk factors. Ramipril had no significant effect on either outcome. In the Nateglinide and Valsartan in Impaired Glucose Tolerance Outcomes Research (NAVIGATOR) study nateglinide had no effect on the progression to diabetes or on cardiovascular outcomes. Valsartan slightly, but significantly, reduced the progression to diabetes, but had no effect on cardiovascular outcomes. Finally, the Canadian Normoglycaemia Outcomes Evaluation (CANOE) trial showed that a low-dose combination of rosiglitazone plus metformin reduced the progression to diabetes, but cardiovascular events were too infrequent to comment upon.

1.4 Insulin resistance and the metabolic syndrome

Insulin resistance (or reduced insulin sensitivity) is established as a key part of type 2 diabetes when combined with beta-cell dysfunction, and more than 90% of patients are insulin resistant. A major advance in the understanding of insulin resistance came with the seminal work of Reaven, who made two key observations:

1. Resistance to insulin-stimulated glucose uptake is present in the majority of patients with impaired glucose tolerance, and type 2 diabetes. He suggested that deterioration of glucose tolerance could only be prevented if the beta-cell is able to increase insulin secretion and maintain chronic hyperinsulinaemia. When this cannot be achieved gross decompensation of glucose homeostasis occurs and diabetes develops.

2. He observed clustering of risk factors for coronary heart disease in individual subjects, including hyperinsulinaemia, impaired glucose tolerance or diabetes, increased plasma triglyceride concentration, decreased HDL cholesterol concentration, and hypertension. He suggested that these might be causally linked by insulin resistance and hyperinsulinaemia, and referred to the cluster as 'Syndrome X'.

Others have referred to this as 'Reaven's syndrome' 'insulin resistance syndrome' or 'metabolic syndrome'. Whether there is a causal link or not, it is clear that insulin resistance is associated with other cardiovascular risk factors such as hyperglycaemia, hypertension and dyslipidaemia. It is unclear why some individuals are insulin resistant, and genetic and environmental factors have both been implicated. In particular physical inactivity and obesity are associated with insulin resistance, but not all obese persons are insulin resistant.

There are several methods of measuring insulin resistance for research purposes, but none are available in routine clinical practice. Several definitions of the metabolic syndrome have been used in the past based on clinical measures and these have recently been harmonized into a joint definition (Table 1.5).

The metabolic syndrome is a strong predictor of subsequent diabetes in non-diabetic individuals. A few studies have shown that

Table 1.5 Criteria for clinical diagnosis of the metabolic syndrome

Measure	Categorical cut points
Elevated waist circumference	Population- and country specific
Elevated triglycerides (drug treatment for elevated trigylerides is an alternate indicator)	≥ 1.7 mmol/L (150 mg/dl)
Reduced HDL-cholesterol (drug treatment for reduced HDL cholesterol is an alternate indicator)	< 1.0 mmol/L (40 mg/dl) in males < 1.3 mmol/L (50 mg/dl) in females
Elevated blood pressure (antihypertensive treatment in a patient with a history of hypertension is an alternate indicator)	Systolic ≥ 130 and/or diastolic ≥ 85 mmHg
Elevated fasting glucose (drug treatment of elevated glucose is an alternate indicator)	≥ 5.6 mmol/L (100 mg/dl)

insulin resistance in patients with type 2 diabetes is associated with increased cardiovascular risk, independent of other risk factors, but this remains controversial.

The metabolic syndrome is not a separate target for treatment in patients with diabetes or in non-diabetic subjects, but the presence of the metabolic syndrome may influence the choice of drugs used for the treatment of hyperglycaemia or hypertension.

1.5 Type 1 diabetes

Prior to the discovery and clinical use of insulin in the 1920s patients with type 1 diabetes survived around one year from the time of diagnosis. Death was caused by infection or severe metabolic acidosis. Initial hopes were that the widespread use of insulin would be a cure for this debilitating and fatal disease. It was soon clear that patients with type 1 diabetes on insulin therapy were surviving, but that their long-term outlook was poor because of the accelerated development of coronary heart disease. The relative risk of the development of coronary heart disease is greatly increased, but as type 1 diabetes affects a younger age group the absolute risk remains low (Figure 1.4).

Because the event rate is lower, and many epidemiological studies combine type 1 and type 2 diabetes, it has been harder to identify what might be cardiovascular risk factors in patients with type 1 diabetes. Observations from the Pittsburgh Epidemiology of Diabetes Complications study have shown associations between incident coronary heart disease events and blood pressure, lipids, white

Figure 1.4 **Coronary heart disease mortality in patients with type 1 diabetes. Data from the Diabetes UK Cohort Study**

Mortality per 100000 per year (log scale)

Age (year)

- --◇-- General, males
- --◆-- Cohort, males
- --△-- General, females
- --▲-- Cohort, females

With kind permission from Springer Science + Business Media: *Diabetologia*. Mortality from heart disease in a cohort of 23,000 patients with insulin-treated diabetes, **46**, 2003, p.762, Laing SP, Swerdlow AJ, Slater SD, *et al.* figure 1.

cell count, renal disease and peripheral vascular disease, with inverse associations with estimated glucose disposal rate and physical activity. Many of these are components of the metabolic syndrome, suggesting that the metabolic syndrome may have an important role in the pathophysiology of cardiovascular disease in type 1 diabetes.

1.6 **Pathology of heart disease in diabetes**

The pathology of coronary heart disease in diabetes is described in Chapter 5. When coronary heart disease develops it is more severe, with more left main stem disease and more triple vessel disease than in non-diabetic subjects, and coronary artery calcification is more extensive. The disease is also more diffuse, affecting proximal and distal segments of an affected artery, which has implications for coronary interventions (see Chapter 7). The development of collateral vessels is also reduced.

In addition to coronary heart disease there is a 'diabetic cardiomyopathy' that can impair systolic emptying or diastolic filling of the left ventricle, and along with coronary heart disease contributes to the high prevalence of chronic heart failure in people with diabetes (Chapter 8).

1.7 **Conclusions**

Cardiovascular disease is a common cause of morbidity and mortality in people with diabetes, and several risk factors for the development

> ## Box 1.1 Interventions to reduce cardiovascular disease in people with type 2 diabetes
>
> Treatment of hyperglycaemia
>
> - Intensive blood glucose control
> - Additional benefits of metformin, pioglitazone.
>
> Treatment of dyslipidaemia
>
> - Statins
> - Additional benefits of high-dose atorvastatin.
>
> Treatment of hypertension
>
> - Multiple antihypertensive drugs
> - Additional benefits of ACE inhibitors, angiotensin II receptor antagonists.
>
> Antiplatelet drugs
>
> - Aspirin and/or clopidogrel for established cardiovascular disease.

of cardiovascular disease in diabetes are identified. There are no randomised control trials or systematic reviews of smoking cessation specifically in people with diabetes, and it is assumed that people with diabetes are likely to benefit from smoking cessation at least as much as people without diabetes. There are now multiple therapies that can be used to reduce cardiovascular risk in people with diabetes (Box 1.1). If we are going to obtain the greatest benefit and wish to reduce polypharmacy we should concentrate on the use of interventions that have a proven evidence base.

References

Alberti KGMM, Eckel RH, Grundy SM, et al. (2009) Harmonizing the metabolic syndrome. *Circulation* **120**: 1640–5.

Bulugahapitiya U, Siyambalapitiya S, Sithole J, Idris I (2009) Is diabetes a coronary risk equivalent? Systematic review and meta-analysis. *Diabetic Medicine* **26**: 142–8.

Chiasson JL, Josse RG, Gomis R, Hanefeld M, Karasik A, Laakso M. For the STOP-NIDDM Trial Research Group (2003) Acarbose treatment and the risk of cardiovascular disease and hypertension in patients with impaired glucose tolerance: the STOP-NIDDM trial. *Journal of the American Medical Association* **290**: 486–94.

Emerging Risk Factors Collaboration (2010) Diabetes mellitus, fasting blood glucose concentration, and risk of vascular disease: a collaborative meta-analysis of 102 prospective studies. *Lancet* **375**: 2215–22.

Evans JM, Wang J, Morris AD (2002) Comparison of cardiovascular risk between patients with type 2 diabetes and those who had had a myocardial infarction: cross sectional and cohort studies. *British Medical Journal* **324**: 939–42.

Haffner SM, Lehto S, Ronnemaa T, Pyorala K, Laakso M (1998) Mortality from coronary heart disease in subjects with type 2 diabetes and in nondiabetic subjects with and without prior myocardial infarction. *New England Journal of Medicine* **339**: 229–34.

Juutilainen A, Lehto S, Ronnemaa T, Pyorala K, Laakso M (2005) Type 2 diabetes as a 'coronary heart disease equivalent': an 18-year prospective population-based study in Finnish subjects. *Diabetes Care* **28**: 2901–7.

Knowler WC, Barrett-Connor E, Fowler SE, *et al.* the Diabetes Prevention Program Research Group (2002) Reduction in the incidence of type 2 diabetes with lifestyle intervention or metformin. *New England Journal of Medicine* **346**: 393–403.

Laing SP, Swerdlow AJ, Slater SD, *et al.* (2003) Mortality from heart disease disease in a cohort of 23,000 patients with insulin-treated diabetes. *Diabetologia* **46**: 760–5.

Reaven GM (1988) Banting lecture 1988 Role of insulin resistance in human disease. *Diabetes* **37**: 1595–607.

Tuomilehto J, Lindstrom J, Eriksson JG, *et al.*, for the Finnish Diabetes Prevention Study Group (2001) Prevention of type 2 diabetes mellitus by changes in lifestyle among subjects with impaired glucose tolerance. *New England Journal of Medicine* **344**: 1343–50.

Chapter 2

Hyperglycaemia and weight management

Miles Fisher

Key points

- Intensive insulin therapy in patients with type 1 diabetes reduces cardiovascular outcomes on long-term follow up
- The treatment of hyperglycaemia in type 2 diabetes reduces cardiovascular events, and on long-term follow up reduces cardiovascular and total mortality. Metformin reduces myocardial infarctions separate from an effect on glycaemia
- Pioglitazone reduces recurrent myocardial infarctions and strokes in type 2 diabetic patients with established cardiovascular disease, but at the expense of increased fluid retention
- Newer antidiabetic drugs have some favourable effects on cardiovascular risk factors
- In patients with type 2 diabetes bariatric surgery reduces weight and leads to remission of diabetes in many patients, with favourable effects on cardiovascular risk factors.

2.1 Management of glycaemia in type 1 diabetes

2.1.1 Diabetes Control and Complications Trial

The Diabetes Control and Complications Trial (DCCT) was established to prove that the intensive control of glycaemia, mimicking the pattern of physiological insulin secretion, reduced diabetic complications in patients with type 1 diabetes. Patients were randomized to intensive insulin therapy administered with an external insulin pump or by three or more daily insulin injections and guided by frequent blood glucose monitoring, or to conventional therapy with one or two daily insulin injections. The patients were followed for a mean of 6.5 years.

Intensive insulin therapy significantly reduced the risk of the development or progression of retinopathy, and reductions were also seen in the occurrence of microalbuminuria, macroalbuminuria, clinical neuropathy, and autonomic neuropathy. The chief adverse events associated with intensive insulin therapy were weight gain and an increase in severe hypoglycaemia.

The effects of intensive insulin therapy in the DCCT on cardiovascular risk factors are described in Box 2.1. The number of combined major cardiovascular events was almost twice as high in the conventionally treated group (40 events) as in the intensive-treatment group (23 events), but the difference was not statistically significant.

2.1.2 Epidemiology of Diabetes Interventions and Complications study

At the end of the DCCT patients were returned to the care of their usual doctor, and patients in the conventional treatment group were offered intensified insulin regimens. Ninety-three per cent of the DCCT subjects were subsequently followed in the observational Epidemiology of Diabetes Interventions and Complications (EDIC) study. The HbA1c concentrations decreased in the group that were formerly conventionally treated, and HbA1c increased in the subjects that were previously intensively treated when they were no

---

Box 2.1 Effects of intensive insulin therapy on cardiovascular risk factors in DCCT

- Reduced fasting, pre-prandial and post-prandial hyperglycaemia
- Reduced HbA1c
- Reduced total and calculated LDL cholesterol
- Reduced triglycerides
- Increased development of low HDL cholesterol (secondary intervention cohort)
- Increased systolic blood pressure
- No difference in diastolic blood pressure
- No difference in smoking habits
- Increased body weight
- Increased development of raised waist-to-hip ratios
- Reduced microalbuminuria
- Reduced macroalbuminuria

longer in the intensive study environment, and thereafter the HbA1c concentrations in the two groups were similar.

During the mean 17 years of total follow-up 46 cardiovascular events occurred in 31 patients who had received intensive treatment in the DCCT, as compared with 98 events in 52 patients who had received conventional treatment. Intensive treatment reduced the risk of any cardiovascular event by 42% and the risk of nonfatal myocardial infarction, stroke, or death from cardiovascular disease by 57% (Figure 2.1). The decrease in HbA1c values during the DCCT was significantly associated with most of the beneficial effects of intensive treatment on the risk of cardiovascular disease, but microalbuminuria and albuminuria also had a role. The pathophysiological mechanisms responsible for the improvements in outcomes and for the prolonged effects of early intervention were unclear, and the authors referred to these as 'metabolic memory'.

Other results of DCCT/EDIC are shown in Box 2.2.

2.1.3 **Cardiovascular effects of hypoglycaemia**
One of the chief adverse events associated with intensive insulin therapy in DCCT was an increase in severe hypoglycaemia, defined as requiring external assistance. Several subgroups defined by baseline characteristics had a particularly high risk of severe hypoglycaemia, including males, adolescents, subjects with no residual C-peptide secretion, and subjects with a previous history of hypoglycaemia. The physical consequences of hypoglycaemia that were reported in the DCCT included coma and seizures, and there were no reported cardiovascular consequences of hypoglycaemia.

Hypoglycaemia provokes an intense counter-regulatory hormonal response, including activation of the autonomic nervous system and the release of epinephrine (adrenaline) and norepinephrine (noradrenaline). The cardiovascular consequences of this include an increase in heart rate, an increase in systolic blood pressure and a decrease in diastolic blood pressure, with widening of the pulse pressure, and an increase in cardiac output. In a patient with coronary heart disease these changes may be enough to cause angina and even myocardial infarction (Box 2.3).

Intensive intravenous insulin treatment may be used to control hyperglycaemia following acute myocardial infarction in diabetic and non-diabetic patients, and hypoglycaemia occurs in one third of patients as a side effect (see p. 72). The changes in pulse and blood pressure are similar, and there are no reports of direct adverse consequences, arrhythmias, or myocardial ischaemia in that particular clinical situation. Some observational data, however, has indicated that hypoglycaemia at the time of presentation with an acute coronary syndrome is associated with a poor prognosis.

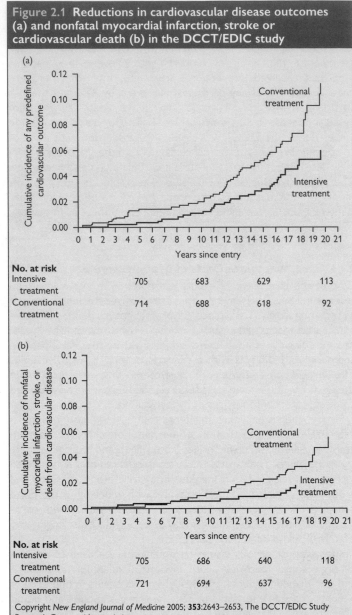

Figure 2.1 **Reductions in cardiovascular disease outcomes (a) and nonfatal myocardial infarction, stroke or cardiovascular death (b) in the DCCT/EDIC study**

Box 2.2 Effects of previous intensive insulin therapy on surrogate markers and endpoints in EDIC

- Reduced progression of retinopathy
- Reduced development and progression of nephropathy
- Reduced neuropathy
- Reduced diabetic autonomic neuropathy
- Reduced incidence of hypertension
- Reduced progression of carotid intima-media thickness (CIMT)
- Reduced coronary artery calcification
- Reduced peripheral arterial calcification
- Lower resting heart rate

Box 2.3 Cardiovascular consequences of hypoglycaemia

Physiological

- Increased heart rate
- Increased systolic blood pressure, decreased diastolic blood pressure, widening of the pulse pressure
- Increased cardiac output
- Decreased peripheral vascular resistance
- Increased left ventricular ejection fraction

Electrocardiography

- Flattening or inversion of the T wave
- Lengthening of the QT interval
- ST segment depression

Arrhythmias

- Atrial and ventricular ectopics
- Sinus bradycardia
- Atrial fibrillation
- Ventricular tachycardia
- Ventricular fibrillation
- Asystole

Pathological

- Silent myocardial ischaemia
- Angina pectoris
- Myocardial infarction
- Cardiac arrest

2.2 Management of glycaemia in type 2 diabetes

2.2.1 Lifestyle measures in type 2 diabetes

Observational studies in diabetic and non-diabetic subjects indicate an association between reduced physical activity and subsequent cardiovascular outcomes. The pathophysiology of type 2 diabetes includes beta-cell dysfunction and insulin resistance. Lifestyle measures, including diet, increased physical activity, and behaviour modification, can reduce insulin resistance and improve glycaemic control and cardiovascular risk markers (reduced HbA1c, reduced systolic and diastolic blood pressure, reduced triglycerides, increased HDL cholesterol, reduced urinary albumin excretion). The ongoing Look AHEAD trial is examining the effects of a lifestyle intervention designed to lose weight on cardiovascular outcomes in people with type 2 diabetes.

2.2.2 Metformin and the United Kingdom Prospective Diabetes Study (UKPDS)

The United Kingdom Prospective Diabetes Study (UKPDS) tested the hypothesis that tight glycaemia control in Type 2 diabetes would reduce microvascular and macrovascular complications, and that there might be advantages with certain agents. This was because an earlier study from the United States had suggested an increase in mortality with the sulphonylurea tolbutamide. The principle comparisons were between a group of patients that received conventional treatment and a group of patients that received intensive treatment based on therapy with a sulphonylurea or insulin. A small subgroup of overweight patients was randomized to metformin.

In the overweight patients metformin significantly reduced myocardial infarctions, cardiovascular deaths and all-cause mortality. The reductions could not be explained by any differences in HbA1c as these were similar in the overweight patients who received intensive treatment with insulin, sulphonylureas and metformin, suggesting that these were due to some other effect of metformin. It was suggested that the beneficial effects of metformin on hepatic insulin resistance or on fibrinolysis might have been responsible for the reduction in myocardial infarctions.

In the intensively treated group tight control reduced microvascular endpoints, in particular the need for photocoagulation for diabetic retinopathy. There was a statistically insignificant reduction in myocardial infarctions during the intervention study.

The main side effects of sulphonylureas in UKPDS were weight gain and hypoglycaemia, and there was no evidence of adverse cardiovascular effects. Sulponylureas and the newer non-sulphonylurea insulin secretagogues repaglinide and nateglinide increase basal and postprandial insulin secretion by closing the K_{ATP} channel in pancreatic beta-cells. In the heart some of these drugs antagonize KATP channels which are important in ischaemic pre- and post-conditioning, and in theory could increase the amount of myocardial damage at the time of myocardial infarction. This has been demonstrated in animal models of infarction and laboratory experiments, but clinical studies have not established a link between sulphonylurea treatment before the acute myocardial infarction and poor outcomes.

Most of the patients in UKPDS were followed in post-trial monitoring for a further ten years. No attempt was made to maintain previously assigned therapies and glycaemic control in the groups rapidly converged, so that between-group differences in HbA1c were lost after the first year. In the group who had received metformin as initial therapy significant reductions in myocardial infarction and all-cause mortality persisted. In the group who had received sulphonylureas or insulin as initial intensive therapy significant reductions in myocardial infarctions and all-cause mortality emerged—a so-called 'legacy' effect (Figure 2.2).

There have been several other publications from the UKPDS that have given useful information about cardiovascular risk in type 2 diabetes (Box 2.4).

2.2.3 Thiazolidinediones or 'glitazones'

The thiazolidinediones rosiglitazone and pioglitazone are agonists for peroxisome-prolferator-activated receptor gamma (PPAR gamma) in adipose tissue, liver and skeletal muscle, reducing insulin resistance and leading to a reduction of blood glucose concentration. When used in man they have potentially beneficial effects on several cardiovascular risk factors (Box 2.5), including reductions in blood pressure and C-reactive protein. Both glitazones cause weight gain. In double blind comparator studies it has been shown that the effects on lipids are different. In particular pioglitazone reduces triglycerides and increases HDL cholesterol, whereas rosiglitazone increases total and LDL cholesterol concentrations.

Glitazones cause the retention of fluid through mechanisms in the distal tubules of the kidney. This may manifest itself as weight gain or ankle oedema. In a patient with early left ventricular systolic function, or diastolic dysfunction, this fluid retention can unmask heart failure. Glitazones are contra-indicated in patients with a history of heart failure (see also Chapter 8).

The PROspective pioglitAzone Clinical Trial In macroVascular Events (PROactive) study examined the effects of pioglitazone on cardiovascular events in patients with type 2 diabetes and existing cardiovascular disease. There was a statistically insignificant reduction of 10% in the primary endpoint, which comprised disease endpoints (death, myocardial infarction, stroke, acute coronary syndromes) and procedural endpoints (coronary revascularization, leg amputation,

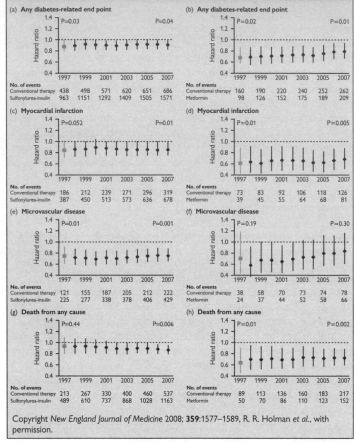

Figure 2.2 Hazard Ratios for any-diabetes related end point, myocardial infarction, microvascular disease, and death from any cause in the UKPDS post-trial monitoring

leg revascularization). A main secondary endpoint of cardiovascular death, myocardial infarction or stroke, was significantly reduced by 16%. Subgroup analysis of patients who had a previous myocardial infarction or strokes showed further reductions in myocardial infarctions and strokes respectively.

One meta-analysis of cardiovascular events in patients treated with pioglitazone demonstrated a significant reduction in all-cause mortality, myocardial infarctions and strokes with pioglitazone in people with type 2 diabetes. Another has shown reduction in all-cause mortality but no effect on non-fatal coronary events. Add Nissen when published (Figure 2.3).

The effects of rosiglitazone on cardiovascular outcomes remain controversial. A meta-analysis was performed of trials where

Box 2.4 Cardiovascular results from the UKPDS

Principal results

- Metformin significantly reduced myocardial infarctions, diabetes-related deaths, and all-cause mortality.

Other important cardiovascular results

- Intensive blood glucose control with metformin was cost-effective in overweight patients with type 2 diabetes.
- The effects of glycaemia and blood pressure reduction on the risk of complications was additive.
- The presence of the metabolic syndrome at baseline identified patients at greater risk of macrovascular but not microvascular complications.
- Insulin sensitivity at diagnosis was not associated with subsequent cardiovascular disease.
- After adjusting for conventional cardiovascular risk factors the risk of myocardial infarction was similar in white and South Asian patients and lower in Afro-Caribbean subjects.

rosiglitazone was given for at least 24 weeks, with a comparable group not receiving rosiglitazone, and the outcome data collected for myocardial infarction and death from cardiovascular causes. In the rosiglitazone group there were 86 myocardial infarctions in 15,560 subjects, and in the comparator group there were 72 myocardial infarctions in 12,283 subjects, giving an odds ratio of 1.43 for myocardial infarction (95% confidence interval 1.03–1.99; $P = 0.03$) with an insignificant increase in cardiovascular deaths. Similar results have been found in an updated meta-analysis from the same authors, and in meta-analyses performed by the Federal Drug Administration (FDA).

Box 2.5 Effects of glitazones on cardiovascular risk factors

Potentially beneficial

- Improved glycaemia control
- Reduced blood pressure
- Reduced microalbuminuria
- Reduced C-reactive protein
- Reduced small dense LDL (especially pioglitazone)
- Increased HDL cholesterol (especially pioglitazone)
- Reduced triglycerides (pioglitazone)

Potentially adverse

- Weight gain
- Increased total and LDL cholesterol (rosiglitazone)

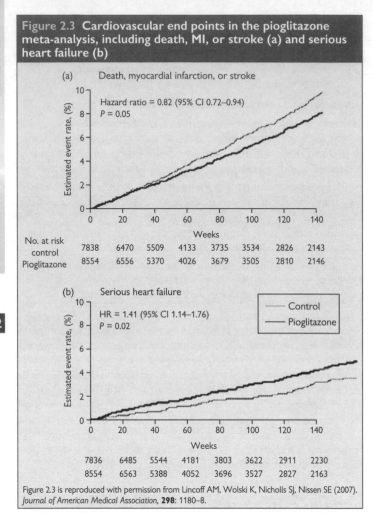

Figure 2.3 **Cardiovascular end points in the pioglitazone meta-analysis, including death, MI, or stroke (a) and serious heart failure (b)**

Figure 2.3 is reproduced with permission from Lincoff AM, Wolski K, Nicholls SJ, Nissen SE (2007). *Journal of American Medical Association*, **298**: 1180–8.

22

The Rosiglitazone Evaluated for Cardiac Outcomes and Regulation of glycaemia in Diabetes (RECORD) study was prospectively established to examine the cardiovascular effects of rosiglitazone. An interim analysis was published following the meta-analysis, which highlighted major deficiencies in study design. The study was open label and not double blind, and was a 'non-inferiority' study. The primary event rate was much lower than predicted. When the RECORD study completed there were no significant differences between the rosiglitazone group and the control group regarding myocardial infarction and death from cardiovascular causes, but an increase in these could not be excluded.

To try and definitively answer safety concerns about rosiglitazone a double-blind trial comparing rosiglitazone with pioglitazone in diabetic patients with vascular disease or high vascular risk was started.

In late 2010 the European Medicines Agency recommended the suspension of marketing authorisation for rosiglitazone across Europe and this has been withdrawn from clinical use.

2.2.4 **Acarbose**

Acarbose is an alpha-glucosidase inhibitor that inhibits digestion of poly-saccharides from the small intestine, reducing post-prandial glucose concentrations. Meta-analysis of the effects of acarbose in patients with type 2 diabetes has given conflicting results. One meta-analysis suggested a reduction in cardiovascular events, whereas a Cochrane review suggested no evidence of any benefit for mortality and morbidity.

2.2.5 **Newer antidiabetic drugs**

Therapies are now available that exploit the incretin effect to treat type 2 diabetes. Glucagon-like peptide 1 (GLP-1) is one of the main incretin hormones, but is rapidly degraded to inactive metabolites by the enzyme dipeptidyl pepitidase-4 (DPP-4). DPP-4 inhibitors are oral drugs that inhibit the action of DPP-4 and increase the amount of endogenous GLP-1 and glucose-dependent insulinotropic peptide (GIP). In clinical use DPP-4 inhibitors reduce HbA1c, have no effect on body weight, and no discernable effect on cardiovascular risk markers.

The alternative approach is to use synthetic agonists of GLP-1 that are resistant to degradation by DPP-4. GLP-1 receptor agonists are given by subcutaneous injection, and increase glucose-dependent promotion of insulin secretion, inhibit glucagon secretion, delay gastric emptying, and suppress appetite, with associated weight loss of 4–5 KGs over one year. This weight loss has in turn been associated with reductions in blood pressure, triglycerides, and increases in HDL cholesterol.

The occurrence of GLP-1 receptors in cardiac tissue and the central nervous system has stimulated investigation of GLP-1 and cardiac effects in animals, but as yet the relevance to humans is uncertain.

Sodium glucose co-transporter 2 inhibitors (SGLT-2 inhibitors) also reduce HbA1c, weight, and blood pressure, which may be related to renal sodium loss. Cardiovascular safety and/or end-point trials are currently in progress with several DPP-4 inhibitors, GLP-1 receptor agonists and SGLT-2 inhibitors.

2.2.6 **Blood glucose targets**

In the UKPDS the mean HbA1c concentration in the intensive treatment group was 7.0%. Two important large multi-centre studies were set up to examine if a lower target HbA1c would reduce cardiovascular events.

The Action in Diabetes and Vascular disease: preterAx and diamicroN-MR Controlled Evaluation (ADVANCE) study aimed to obtain a target HbA1c of 6.5% in the intensive group, and this was achieved 3 years into the study. There was a significant reduction in microvascular events with more intensive therapy in ADVANCE, but no significant effect, either beneficial or harmful, on macrovascular events

Figure 2.4 Probability of events of non-fatal myocardial infarction with intensive glucose-lowering versus standard treatment (Ray et al., 2009)

	Intensive treatment/ standard treatment		Weight of study size	Odds ratio (95% CI)	Odds ratio (95% CI)
	Participants	Events			
UKPDS[4,7]	3071/1549	221/141	21.8%		0.78 (0.62–0.98)
PROactive[18–20]	2605/2633	119/144	18.0%		0.83 (0.64–1.06)
ADVANCE[5]	5571/5569	153/156	21.9%		0.98 (0.78–1.23)
VADT[21,22]	892/899	64/78	9.4%		0.81 (0.58–1.15)
ACCORD[8]	5128/5123	186/235	28.9%		0.78 (0.64–0.95)
Overall	17267/15773	743/754	100%		0.83 (0.75–0.93)

0.4   0.6   0.8   1.0   1.2 1.4 1.6 1.8 2.0

Intensive treatment better   Standard treatment better

Reprinted from *The Lancet*, **373**, Kausik K Ray, Sreenivasa Rao Kondapally Seshasai, Shanelle Wijesuriya, Rupa Sivakumaran, Sarah Nethercott, David Preiss, Sebhat Erqou, Naveed Sattar. Effect of intensive control of glucose on cardiovascular outcomes and death in patients with diabetes mellitus: a meta-analysis of randomised controlled trials, 1765–1772. Copyright (2009), with permission from Elsevier.

or mortality. Weight gain and hypoglycaemia were not common in ADVANCE.

The Action to Control Cardiovascular Risk in Diabetes (ACCORD) study aimed to reduce HbA1c rapidly to non-diabetic levels. The target HbA1c of less than 6.0% was not reached because of severe hypoglycaemia and marked weight gain, and a level of 6.5% was obtained by six months. The study was stopped early because of an increase in total mortality in the intensive treatment group. To date the investigators have failed to explain the increased mortality. As several of the deaths were sudden or unexpected, undetected hypoglycaemia provoking arrhythmias is one possible explanation.

Several meta-analyses have been performed which have included data from UKPDS, ADVANCE and ACCORD. Significant reductions in myocardial infarctions and coronary events have been observed, with no significant effect on cardiovascular or total mortality (Figure 2.4). The target HbA1c for the prevention of cardiovascular disease in diabetes should be less than 7.0% and not lower than 6.5%.

2.3 Weight loss and cardiovascular outcomes

2.3.1 Principles of drug therapy for obesity

Anti-obesity agents can have indirect effects on insulin resistance and hyperglycaemia mediated by weight loss. Treatments include drugs that decrease nutrient absorption, and drugs that decrease food intake by reducing appetite or increasing satiety. Appetite suppressants work by changing the availability of neurotransmitters. In the past noradrenergic agents were used, but are no longer recommended because of the risk of abuse. Fenfluramine, a drug that stimulated the release of serotonin and inhibited its reuptake, was withdrawn because of associations with valvular heart disease and pulmonary hypertension.

Rimonabant was an appetite suppressant that promoted weight loss through blockade of the type 1 cannabinoid receptor. In diabetic patients the use of this agent was associated with increased weight loss, reductions in HbA1c, improvements in lipids, and reductions in blood pressure. The main side effect was an increase in depression and suicidal ideation, and the drug was withdrawn because of this.

Sibutramine inhibits the reuptake of norepinephrine and serotonin, promoting satiety and weight loss. When used in type 2 diabetes it promotes reductions in HbA1c and triglycerides, with an increase in HDL cholesterol, and no change in total and LDL cholesterol. Sibutramine can substantially increase pulse and blood pressure in some patients. Results from the Sibutramine Cardiovascular Outcomes Trial (SCOUT) showed an increase in serious, non-fatal cardiovascular events which led to suspension of the drug in Europe.

2.3.2 **Orlistat**

Orlistat is a gastric and pancreatic lipase inhibitor that reduces dietary fat absorption, and when used in addition to other antidiabetic drugs, including metformin, sulphonylureas and insulin, has resulted in increased weight loss and a reduction in HbA1c, blood pressure, total and LDL cholesterol, with a slight reduction in HDL cholesterol.

2.3.3 **Bariatric surgery**

A variety of surgical procedures now exist that cause weight reduction. Procedures can be grouped into purely restrictive, mostly restrictive and mostly malabsorptive. The least invasive procedure is laparoscopic adjustable gastric banding (LAGB). Bilio-pancreatic diversion (BPD) is the most invasive of the procedures and carries the greatest peri-operative risk, but in the longer term has the potential for greater weight loss.

Bariatric surgery has been demonstrated to improve glycaemic control and in many patients with a short duration of disease to result in remission from diabetes. Significant improvements or resolution of hypertension, dyslipidaemia and sleep apnoe have also been demonstrated. Relatively little is know about the long-term effects of bariatric surgery on cardiovascular morbidity and mortality. Observational data from a cohort study in Sweden has shown a long-term reduction in mortality compared to obese patients that did not get bariatric surgery.

References

Action to Control Cardiovascular Risk in Diabetes Study Group (2008) Effects of intensive glucose lowering in type 2 diabetes. *New England Journal of Medicine* **358**: 2545–59.

ADVANCE Collaborative Group (2008) Intensive blood glucose control and vascular outcomes in patients with type 2 diabetes. *New England Journal of Medicine* **358**: 2560–72.

Diabetes Control and Complications Trial (DCCT) Research Group (1995) Effect of intensive diabetes management on macrovascular events and risk factors in the Diabetes Control and Complications Trial. *American Journal of Cardiology* **75**, 894–903.

Diabetes Control and Complications Trial/Epidemiology of Diabetes Interventions and Complications (DCCT/EDIC) Study Research Group (2005) Intensive diabetes treatment and cardiovascular disease in patients with type 1 diabetes. *New England Journal of Medicine* **353**: 2643–53.

Dormandy JA, Charbonnel B, Eckland DJA, *et al.* on behalf of the PROactive investigators. (2005) Secondary prevention of macrovascular events in patients with type 2 diabetes in the PROactive study (PROspective pioglitAzone Clinical Trial in macroVascular Events): a randomised controlled trial. *Lancet* **366**: 1279–89.

Holman RR, Paul SK, Bethel MA, Mathews DR, Neil HAW (2008) 10-year follow-up of intensive blood glucose control in type 2 diabetes. *New England Journal of Medicine* **359**: 1577–89.

Lincoff AM, Wolski K, Nicholls SJ, Nissen SE (2007) Pioglitazone and risk of cardiovascular events in patients with type 2 diabetes mellitus: a meta-analysis of randomized trials. *Journal of the American Medical Association* **298**, 1180–8.

Nissen SE, Wolski K (2007) Effect of rosiglitazone on the risk of myocardial infarction and death from cardiovascular causes. *New England Journal of Medicine* **356**: 2457–71.

Nissen SE, Wolski K (2010) Rosiglitazone revisited: an updated meta-analysis for risk of myocardial infarction and cardiovascular mortality. *Archives of Internal Medicine* **170**: 1191–201.

Ray KK, Seshasai SRK, Wijesuriya S, *et al.* (2009) Effect of intensive control of glucose on cardiovascular outcomes and death in patients with diabetes mellitus: a meta-analysis of randomised controlled trials. *Lancet* **373**: 1765–72.

UK Prospective Diabetes Study (UKPDS) Group (1998a) Intensive blood-glucose control with sulphonylureas or insulin compared with conventional treatment and risk of complications in patients with type 2 diabetes (UKPDS 33). *Lancet* **352**: 837–53.

UK Prospective Diabetes Study (UKPDS) Group (1998b) Effect of intensive blood-glucose control with metformin on complications in overweight patients with type 2 diabetes (UKPDS 34). *Lancet* **352**: 854–65.

Chapter 3

Diabetic dyslipidaemia

Miles Fisher

Key points

- The typical dyslipidaemia in type 2 diabetes and the metabolic syndrome comprises low HDL cholesterol concentrations and raised triglycerides. Total and LDL cholesterol are not raised, but the proportion of atherogenic small-dense LDL cholesterol is increased
- In large studies statins have been proven to reduce cardiovascular events in people with diabetes who have known cardiovascular disease ('secondary prevention') and who have increased cardiovascular risk ('primary prevention')
- Larger doses of statins have further reduced cardiovascular events in people with cardiovascular disease and diabetes compared to smaller doses, but with an increase in side-effects
- Few studies have included patients with type 1 diabetes, and the clinical use of statins in patients with type 1 diabetes, and in younger patients with type 2 diabetes, is based on extrapolation from older patients with type 2 diabetes
- Fibrates reduce triglycerides and increase HDL cholesterol, but the results of large studies with fibrates in patients with diabetes have been disappointing and mostly negative.

3.1 Description of the dyslipidaemia of diabetes

Diabetes and dyslipidaemia are components of the metabolic syndrome. The typical dyslipdaemia of diabetes consists of low HDL cholesterol concentrations, raised triglycerides, and an increase in the proportion of small dense particles of LDL cholesterol, which

Box 3.1 Diabetic dyslipidaemia
Increased
• Triglycerides
• Apolipoprotein B
• Very low density lipoproteins (VLDLs), especially VLDL1
• Triglyceride-rich remnants
• Small dense LDL
• Postprandial lipaemia.
Decreased
• HDL cholesterol, especially HDL2
• Apolipoprotein A-1.

are more atherogenic than larger LDL particles. There are associated abnormalities in other lipid sub-fractions and apolipoproteins (Box 3.1).

Epidemiolgical evidence has shown a strong association between levels of total and LDL cholesterol and vascular events, an inverse relationship between HDL concentrations and vascular events, and in some epidemiological studies raised triglycerides were a risk factor for vascular events independent of low HDL concentrations. Of the available lipid-regulating drugs fibrates improve the lipid profile, reducing triglycerides and increasing HDL cholesterol, but there is limited evidence from clinical trials that this reduces cardiovascular events, and most of the evidence is for statins.

3.2 **Statins**

Statins competitively inhibit 3-hydroy-3-methylglutaryl A (HMG CoA) reductase, reducing cholesterol synthesis in the liver. There is evidence of cardiovascular risk reduction with statins in people with diabetes, both as primary and secondary prevention, and for several different statins, suggesting a possible class-effect (Box 3.2).

Not every study has been positive, and there are studies where the benefit in people with diabetes has not reached statistical significance, possibly because of small numbers in the subgroup. In one study in older patients the number of events was insignificantly increased in diabetic subjects treated with pravastatin compared to diabetic patients treated with placebo, although the study overall showed significant cardiovascular benefit from pravastatin.

3.2.1 **Older statins—simvastatin and pravastatin**
Initial statin trials were in patients with established coronary heart disease and raised total cholesterols, using simvastatin and pravastatin.

Box 3.2 Evidence for benefits of statins in diabetic patients

Statins of proven benefit

- Stable coronary disease (simvastatin, pravastatin, atorvastatin)
- Patients without known vascular disease ('primary prevention') (simvastatin, atorvastatin)
- Acute coronary syndromes (atorvastatin)
- Following coronary artery bypass surgery (lovastatin)
- Following percutaneous coronary interventions (fluvastatin)
- Following stroke (simvastatin, atorvastatin)
- Chronic kidney disease (CKD) (pravastatin, atorvastatin).

Statin studies negative

- Chronic renal failure
- Haemodialysis patients
- Chronic heart failure.

Subgroup analysis of diabetic subgroups demonstrated similar relative risk reductions for total mortality, cardiovascular mortality and major coronary events, and as the event rate was higher in people with diabetes the absolute risk reduction was greater.

The Scandinavian Simvastatin Survival Study (4S) examined the effects of simvastatin in patients with angina or previous myocardial infarction and raised total cholesterol. Most patients received 20 mg of simvastatin, but around one third had the dose increased to 40 mg. Simvastatin reduced the primary endpoint of total mortality, and there was a significant reduction in 'major coronary events' (coronary heart disease related death and non-fatal MI). There were two post-hoc subgroup analyses of diabetic patients. The first examined patients with known diabetes at the start of the study, and revealed significant reductions in major coronary events. The second added people diagnosed using the WHO 1999 criteria, and the reduction in major coronary events was similar. There have been several other publications from 4S that have given useful information about cardiovascular risk in type 2 diabetes (Box 3.3).

Results similar to 4S were found using pravastatin for secondary prevention in the Cholesterol and Recurrent Events (CARE) trial and the Long-Term Intervention with Pravastatin in Ischaemic Disease (LIPID) trial. The West of Scotland Coronary Prevention Study (WOSCOPS) with pravastatin was the first study to demonstrate reduced cardiovascular events in subjects without myocardial infarction, but WOSCOPS contained only 76 known diabetic patients (1%) so subgroup analysis of diabetic patients was not possible.

Later statin trials were performed in subjects with 'normal' cholesterol concentrations, patients with other forms of vascular disease,

> ### Box 3.3 Results of the 4S study
>
> **Principal results**
>
> - In patients with diabetes and coronary heart disease simvastatin significantly reduced major coronary heart disease events and insignificantly reduced total mortality.
>
> **Other results from 4S**
>
> - For patients with diabetes estimates of cost per life-year gained were well within the range generally considered to be cost effective.
> - In patients with impaired fasting glucose simvastatin reduced major coronary events, revascularizations, total and coronary mortality.
> - Simvastatin significantly reduced cardiovascular disease-related hospitalizations and total hospital days for patients with normal fasting glucose, impaired fasting glucose and diabetes, and significantly reduced length of stay for people with diabetes.
> - Non-diabetic patients with or without the metabolic syndrome benefited from simvastatin. The absolute benefit was greater in patients with the metabolic syndrome because they had a higher absolute risk.

and diabetic patients without known vascular disease. The Heart Protection Study (HPS) addressed the possible benefit of simvastatin 40 mg in 20 536 subjects who would not have been included in the early coronary studies. There were 5,963 diabetic subjects (29% of the total), mostly with type 2 diabetes. This was the first study to demonstrate a reduction in strokes with statins in addition to the reduction in coronary events in people with diabetes (Figure 3.1). 2912 diabetic patients (49% of diabetic subjects) had no prior occlusive vascular disease (primary prevention), and simvastatin significantly reduced the primary endpoint of first major cardiovascular event from 13% down to 9% in this sub-group.

Of the older statins, there is a large evidence base for the use of simvastatin and pravastatin for both primary and secondary prevention in people with diabetes.

Lovastatin and fluvastatin have been shown to be of benefit in diabetic patients following coronary artery bypass grafting and percutaneous coronary interventions (Box 3.2). Together these results suggest that the benefits of statins are a probably a class-effect.

3.2.2 Newer statins—atorvastatin

Atorvastatin is the only one of the newer, more potent statins that has been proven in large, placebo controlled endpoint studies. The Collaborative AtoRvastatin Diabetes Study (CARDS) was the first

Figure 3.1 Reductions in vascular events with simvastatin 40 mg in people with and without diabetes in the Heart Protection Study (HPS)

Major vascular event and prior disease group	Simvastatin-allocated (10 269)	Placebo-allocated (10 267)	Event rate ratio (95% CI)		P-value for heterogeneity
Major coronary events					
Diabetes	279 (9.4%)	377 (12.6%)			
No diabetes	619 (8.5%)	335 (11.5%)			
Subtotal: coronary event	898 (8.7%)	1212 (11.8%)	0.73 (0.67–0.79) P<0.0001		1.0
Strokes					
Diabetes	149 (5.0%)	193 (6.5%)			
No diabetes	295 (4.0%)	392 (5.4%)			
Subtotal: stroke	444 (4.3%)	585 (5.7%)	0.75 (0.66–0.85) P<0.0001		0.9
Revascularizations					
Diabetes	260 (8.7%)	309 (10.4%)			
No diabetes	679 (9.3%)	896 (12.3%)			
Subtotal: revascularization	939 (9.1%)	1205 (11.7%)	0.76 (0.70–0.83) P<0.0001		0.3
Major vascular events					
Diabetes	601 (20.2%)	748 (25.1%)			
No diabetes	1432 (19.6%)	1837 (25.2%)			
Any major vascular event	2033 (19.8%)	2585 (25.2%)	0.76 (0.72–0.81) P<0.0001		0.6

Simvastatin better   Placebo better

0.6   0.8   1.0   1.2   1.4

Reprinted from *The Lancet*, **361**, Heart Protection Study Collaborative Group, MRC/BHF Heart Protection Study of cholesterol-lowering with simvastatin in 5963 people with diabetes: a randomised placebo-controlled trial, 2005-16. Copyright (2003), with permission from Elsevier.

study which assessed the benefits of cholesterol reduction solely in a cohort of subjects with diabetes, and randomised 2838 participants with type 2 diabetes and no previous cardiovascular disease to atorvastatin 10 mg or placebo.

CARDS was stopped early because of a significant reduction of 37% in the composite primary endpoint of 'major cardiovascular events', which comprised all acute coronary heart disease events including resuscitated cardiac arrest, coronary revascularization procedures and stroke. The largest benefit was seen in stroke prevention with a 48% risk reduction. These results were seen with initial LDL levels both above and below the median. Further analysis of the data showed that atorvastatin was cost effective, significantly reduced major cardiovascular events as early as 18 months after initiation of treatment with a significant reduction in coronary heart disease events as early as one year, and was effective in patients aged 65–75 years.

3.2.3 **Rosuvastatin**

Rosuvastatin is a newer, more potent statin, which causes greater reductions in total and LDL cholesterol. There are no endpoint trials to support rosuvastatin use in people with diabetes, and it should be considered where diabetic patients have failed to reach targets with one of the other statins. In the Justification for the Use of statins in Prevention: an Intervention Trial Evaluating Rosuvastatin (JUPITER) study rosuvastatin reduced cardiovascular events in subjects with a low LDL cholesterol and high concentrations of CRP, but people with diabetes were excluded. Indeed, there was a slight but significant increase in the development of new diabetes in subjects given rosuvastatin, which has been confirmed in meta-analysis of trials with all statins. Rosuvastatin should be considered where diabetic patients have failed to reach targets with one of the other statins (Table 3.1).

3.2.4 **Ezetimibe**

An alternative approach if the patient fails to reach target is the addition of ezetimibe. Ezetimibe is a cholesterol absorption inhibitor so has a mode of action that is complementary to statins. It has been shown to lead to substantial reductions in cholesterol when added to statins in patients with diabetes. To date several double-blind, randomized endpoint trials with ezetimibe have been negative. However, a trial in patients with chronic kidney disease, one quarter of whom had diabetes, demonstrated reductions in major vascular events, and a trial in patients following acute coronary syndromes is in progress.

3.2.5 **Higher doses of statins**

Observations have suggested that lower total or LDL cholesterol concentrations are associated with lower vascular events rates,

Table 3.1 Lipid lowering therapy in diabetes

	Primary prevention	Secondary prevention
Which patients?	All patients >40 years of age, high risk <40 years	All diabetic patients
Which statin?	Simvastatin 40 mg, or atorvastatin 10 mg	Simvastatin 40 mg, atorvastatin 80 mg if acute coronary syndrome
What total cholesterol target?	<5.0 mmol/l	<4.0 mmol/l
What LDL cholesterol target?	<3.0 mmol/l	<2.0 mmol/l
What to do if not to target?	Switch to more potent statin e.g. atorvastatin 40 mg, or add ezetimibe 10 mg	Switch to more potent statin e.g. atorvastatin 80 mg, or add ezetimibe 10 mg

leading to the hypothesis that higher doses of statins, causing greater reductions in cholesterol, would lead to greater reductions in vascular events. Most of the comparisons have used high-dose atorvastatin, and further reductions in cardiovascular events have been demonstrated, including in diabetic subgroups. This has included in patients with acute coronary syndromes, stable coronary heart disease, and strokes.

The Pravastatin or Atorvastatin Evaluation and Infection Therapy-Thrombolysis in Myocardial Infraction 22 (PROVE-IT TIMI 22) trial compared 40 mg of pravastatin versus 80 mg of atorvastatin in patients with recent acute coronary syndromes. At the start of the study they had modestly elevated total and LDL cholesterol levels of 4.7 and 2.7 mmol/l respectively. After a mean follow up period of 24 months the atorvastatin group achieved a 32% reduction in LDL cholesterol (2.7 to 1.6 mmol/l) compared to minor reductions seen with pravastatin (2.7 to 2.4 mmol/l). There was a 16% reduction in the primary endpoint of time to first major cardiovascular event, including death from any cause, MI, unstable angina, stroke, and revascularization procedures. There were 978 subjects with diabetes in the study (23%). There was a non-significant reduction in the time to first major cardiovascular event within this subgroup probably reflecting the relatively small number of patients with diabetes. Acute coronary events were significantly reduced by 25% (Figure 3.2).

The Treatment to New Targets (TNT) study looked at atorvastatin 10 mg versus 80 mg in patients with stable coronary heart disease. This was a large, open label study which randomised 10,001

Figure 3.2 Reductions in death, myocardial infarction and unstable angina in patients with diabetes and non-diabetic subjects in the PROVE IT trial

□ Pravastatin 40 mg   ■ Atorvastatin 80 mg

HR (95% CI)
DM   0.75 (0.58–0.97), P = 0.03
No DM   0.76 (0.64–0.90), P = 0.002

Diabetes (n = 978): 26.6, 21.1
No diabetes (n = 3184): 18, 14
Event rate (%)

patients with coronary heart disease, 15% of whom had diabetes. By the end of the run in period the mean LDL in both patient groups was 2.6 mmol/l. This was reduced further to a mean of 2.0 mmol/l in the 80 mg atorvastatin group and resulted in a significant 22% relative risk reduction in the primary endpoint of major cardiovascular events, which included death from coronary heart disease or stroke, non-fatal or procedural MI, resuscitated cardiac arrest or non-fatal stroke.

In diabetic subjects there was a 25% relative risk reduction in major cardiovascular events, which was seen for all quintiles of age, initial LDL or duration of diabetes and in patients with HbA1c < or > 7% (Figure 3.3). A marked reduction was particularly demonstrated in diabetic patients with chronic kidney disease. There were too few subjects to see significant reductions in most of the secondary endpoints although there was a significant reduction in the time to cerebrovascular events and time to cardiovascular events with high dose atorvastatin.

In both PROVE IT and TNT the main side effect of higher dose statins was an increase in abnormalities of liver function tests.

3.2.6 **Systematic reviews and meta-analyses**

There are several systematic reviews and meta-analyses of statin studies in people with diabetes. In one meta-analysis comparing diabetic and non-diabetic subjects it was demonstrated that lipids were reduced to a similar degree in both groups, but that diabetic patients

Figure 3.3 Further reductions in cardiovascular events in people with diabetes in the Treating to New Targets (TNT) study

benefited more in both primary and secondary prevention because of the greater absolute risk reduction.

The Cholesterol Treatment Trialists' (CTT) Collaborators performed a meta-analysis of cholesterol-lowering therapy in 18 686 people with diabetes in 14 randomized trials of statins. There was a 9% reduction in all-cause mortality per mmol/L reduction in LDL cholesterol, with a 21% reduction in major vascular events per mmol/L reduction in LDL cholesterol. There was some limited direct evidence of benefit in 1466 people with type 1 diabetes (Figure 3.4).

3.2.7 Statins for lower-risk diabetic patients

There were very few subjects with type 1 diabetes in the studies described above, and most subjects were middle-aged or elderly. Many guidelines suggest the use of statins in younger patients with diabetes, and suggest ways of identifying younger patients with diabetes who are at increased risk. These include using formal risk calculation, or use in patients with components of the metabolic syndrome (low HDL cholesterol, raised triglycerides, hypertension) a family history of CVD, retinopathy, or nephropathy.

3.2.8 Cholesterol targets in diabetes

Several different targets are set in different guidelines for cholesterol lowering in people with diabetes. Some include an 'audit' total cholesterol of 5 mmol/l, and an LDL cholesterol of 3 mmol/l.

Figure 3.4 Effects on major vascular events per mmol/L reduction in LDL cholesterol by baseline factors in the CTT Collaboration

Groups	Events (%) Treatment	Events (%) Control		RR (CI)	Test for heterogenity or trend
Type of diabetes:					
Type 1 diabetes:	147 (20.5%)	196 (26.2%)		0.79 (0.62–1.01)	χ^2_1=0.0; p=1.0
Type 2 diabetes:	1318 (15.2%)	1586 (18.5%)		0.79 (0.72–0.87)	
Sex:					
Men	1082 (17.2%)	1332 (21.4%)		0.78 (0.71–0.86)	χ^2_1=0.1; p=0.7
Women	383 (12.4%)	450 (14.6%)		0.81 (0.67–0.97)	
Age (years):					
≤65	701 (13.1%)	898 (17.1%)		0.77 (0.68–0.87)	χ^2_1=0.5; p=0.5
>65	764 (18.9%)	884 (21.8%)		0.81 (0.71–0.92)	
Currently treated hypertension:					
Yes	1030 (16.3%)	1196 (19.1%)		0.82 (0.74–0.91)	χ^2_1=2.7; p=0.1
No	435 (14.2%)	586 (19.3%)		0.73 (0.63–0.85)	
Body-mass index:					
<25.0	276 (15.7%)	362 (20.4%)		0.78 (0.64–0.95)	
225.0–<30.0	639 (15.9%)	774 (18.9%)		0.77 (0.68–0.88)	χ^2_1=0.5; p=0.5
230.0	532 (15.1%)	628 (17.6%)		0.82 (0.71–0.95)	
Systolic blood pressure (mmHg):					
<160	993 (15.0%)	1276 (19.1%)		0.76 (0.69–0.85)	χ^2_1=1.3; p=0.3
≥160	472 (17.1%)	505 (19.2%)		0.83 (0.71–0.96)	
Diastolic blood pressure (mmHg):					
≤90	1176 (16.5%)	1417 (19.8%)		0.81 (0.73–0.89)	χ^2_1=1.7; p=0.2
>90	288 (12.9%)	364 (17.1%)		0.73 (0.61–0.87)	
Smoking status:					
Current smokers	266 (17.5%)	347 (22.5%)		0.78 (0.64–0.96)	χ^2_1=0.0; p=0.9
Non-smokers	1199 (15.2%)	1435 (18.5%)		0.79 (0.72–0.87)	
Estimated GFR(mL/min/1.73m²):					
<60	415 (20.6%)	477 (24.0%)		0.83 (0.71–0.97)	
260–<90	816 (15.5%)	961 (18.4%)		0.81 (0.72–0.91)	χ^2_1=2.9; p=0.09
290	194 (12.5%)	286 (18.7%)		0.65 (0.50–0.84)	
Predicted risk of major vascular event (per year):					
<4.5%	474 (8.4%)	631 (11.2%)		0.74 (0.64–0.85)	
24.5%–<8.0%	472 (23.2%)	540 (27.3%)		0.80 (0.66–0.96)	χ^2_1=1.8; p=0.2
28.0%	519 (30.5%)	611 (35.8%)		0.82 (0.70–0.95)	
All diabetes	**1465 (15.6%)**	**1782 (19.2%)**		**0.79 (0.74–0.84)**	

Global test for heterogeneity within subtotals: χ^2_{13}=13.9; p=0.4
0.5   1.0   1.5
■ RR (99% CI)
◇ RR (95% CI)
Treatment better   Control better

Reprinted from *The Lancet*, **371**, Cholesterol Treatment Trialists' (CTT) Collaborators, Efficacy of cholesterol-lowering therapy in 18 686 people with diabetes in 14 randmosied trials of statins: a meta-analysis, 117-125. Copyright (2008), with permission from Elsevier.

Scientific evidence supports the use of higher-dose statins to lower targets of 4 mmol/l total cholesterol and 2 mmol/l LDL cholesterol. This approach is strongly recommended for patients with established cardiovascular disease, especially following acute coronary syndromes.

3.3 Other lipid lowering drugs

3.3.1 Fibrates

Fibrates act through PPAR alpha, leading to increases in HDL cholesterol and reductions in triglycerides. In theory they should be more suitable to correct the dyslipidaemia of diabetes and reduce cardiovascular events, but the evidence for this is rather limited. Several of the clinical trails of fibrates in diabetes have been negative, and only gemfibrozil is of clearly proven benefit in diabetic patients with coronary heart disease. Other studies have shown benefits with statins in similar groups of patients, and combination of gemfibrozil with a statin is contraindicated because of an increase in muscle side effects.

The Fenofibrate Intervention and Event Lowering in Diabetes (FIELD) study examined the effects of fenofibrate in people with diabetes, mostly without existing vascular disease. There was no effect of fenofibrate on the main endpoint of cardiovascular death and myocardial infarction. Post-hoc analysis demonstrated some reductions in other endpoints in subgroups. Further analysis from the FIELD study has shown a significant reduction in microalbuminuria and diabetic retinopathy. The mechanism for this is unknown, and further research is required.

The ACCORD study included a lipid arm where fenofibrate or placebo was added in combination with simvasatin. No significant reduction was seen in any of the cardiovascular events.

A recent meta-analysis, including data from FIELD has demonstrated that fibrates as a class reduce cardiovascular outcomes. Subgroup analysis for coronary events showed no significant benefit in patients with diabetes.

3.4 Conclusions

The use of statins is now a routine part of the management of middle-aged and elderly diabetic patients. Serious consideration should be given to using high-dose statins in patients with existing cardiovascular disease, especially following acute coronary syndromes.

References

Ahmed S, Cannon CP, Murphy SA, Braunwald E (2006) Acute coronary syndromes and diabetes: is intensive lipid lowering beneficial? Results of the PROVE IT-TIMI 22 trial. *European Heart Journal* **27**; 2323–9.

Cholesterol Trialists' (CTT) Collaborators (2008) Efficacy of cholesterol-lowering therapy in 18 686 people with diabetes in 14 randomised trials of statins: a meta-analysis. *Lancet* **371**: 117–25.

Colhoun HM, Betteridge DJ, Durrington PN, *et al.* on behalf of the CARDS investigators (2004) Primary prevention of cardiovascular disease with atrovastatin in type 2 diabetes in the Collaborative Atorvastatin Diabetes Study (CARDS): multicentre randomised placebo-controlled trial. *Lancet* **364**: 685–96.

Costa J, Borges M, David C, Vaz Carneiro A (2006) Efficacy of lipid lowering drug treatment for diabetic and non-diabetic patients: meta-analysis of randomised controlled trails. *British Medical Journal* **332**: 1115–24.

Field Study Investigators (2005) Effects of long-term fenofibrate therapy on cardiovascular events in 9795 people with type 2 diabetes (the FIELD study): randomised controlled trial. *Lancet* **366**: 1849–61.

Goldberg RB, Mellies MJ, Sacks FM, et al. for the CARE Investigators (1998) Cardiovascular events and their reduction with pravastatin in diabetic and glucose-intolerant myocardial infarction survivors with average cholesterol levels. Subgroup analyses in the Cholesterol And Recurrent Events (CARE) Trial. *Circulation* **98**: 2513–9.

Heart Protection Study Collaborative Group (2003) MRC/BHF Heart Protection Study of cholesterol-lowering with simvastatin in 5963 people with diabetes: a randomised placebo-controlled trial. *Lancet* **361**: 2005–16.

Keech A, Colquhoun D, Best J, et al. for the LIPID Study Group (2003) Secondary prevention of cardiovascular events with long-term pravastatin in patients with diabetes or impaired fasting glucose: results from the LIPID trial. *Diabetes Care* **26**: 2713–21.

Pyorala K, Pedersen TR, Kjekshus J, Faergeman O, Olsson AG, Thorgeirsson G, and the Scandinavian Simvastatin Survival Study (4S) Group (1997) Cholesterol lowering with simvastatin improves prognosis of diabetic patients with coronary heart disease. A subgroup analysis of the Scandinavian Simvastatin Survival Study (4S). *Diabetes Care* **20**: 614–20.

Shepherd J, Barter P, Carmena R, et al. for the Treating to New Targets Investigators (2006) Effect of lowering LDL cholesterol substantially below currently recommended levels in patients with coronary heart disease and diabetes: the Treating to New Targets (TNT) study. *Diabetes Care* **29**: 1220–6.

Chapter 4

Hypertension in diabetes

Miles Fisher

Key points

- Hypertension is common in patients with type 2 diabetes and is a component of the metabolic syndrome
- Aggressive treatment of hypertension in patients with type 2 diabetes reduces microvascular complications, strokes, myocardial infarctions, and total mortality
- The greatest benefit is obtained by aggressive lowering of blood pressure, and the choice of antihypertensive drug is a secondary consideration
- Older antihypertensive agents may be less effective than newer agents in lowering blood pressure, and angiotensin-converting enzyme inhibitors and angiotensin-II receptor antagonists may have some advantages in further reducing acute cardiovascular events and diabetic nephropathy
- Targets for blood pressure lowering are lower in people with diabetes, and to achieve these targets requires the use of multiple antihypertensive drugs.

4.1 Mechanisms of hypertension in diabetes

Hypertension is common in patients with diabetes. In patients with type 1 diabetes blood pressure is slightly increased compared to age-matched non-diabetic control subjects. Blood pressure increases further in type 1 patients who have microalbuminuria, and hypertension is common in patients with macroalbuminuria (see also Chapter 10).

Hypertension is very common in people with type 2 diabetes, is two-three times more common than in the age-matched general population, and is a component of the metabolic syndrome. Obese people have a greater risk of hypertension. For each unit increase in body mass index the prevalence of hypertension increases

> **Box 4.1 Possible mechanisms of hypertension with insulin resistance**
>
> • Insulin-stimulated sodium and water retention through the distal renal tubules
> • Increased contractility and vascular resistance
> • Increased sympathetic stimulation
> • Vascular smooth muscle proliferation
> • Impaired insulin-mediated vasodilation

by 1.0–1.5%. There are several possible explanations for the link between insulin resistance and hypertension (Box 4.1).

Untreated hypertension in diabetes increases the risk of cardio-vascular disease (myocardial infarction, congestive cardiac failure, stroke) and microvascular disease (retinopathy, nephropathy).

If a definition of hypertension of a blood pressure greater than 140/90 mmHg is adopted, then at least 40% of patients with type 2 diabetes will have hypertension. It should be noted that the risk of vascular events in people with diabetes increases even within the normal range i.e. blood pressure is a continuous risk factor. Evidence from the Action in Diabetes and Vascular disease: preterAx and dia-microN-MR Controlled Evaluation (ADVANCE) study shows that reduction of blood pressure in diabetic patients with a 'normal' blood pressure i.e. less that 140/90 mmHg will reduce events (See 4.2.3).

There are several endocrine diseases where diabetes and hyper-tension are both present, including Cushing's syndrome, phaeochro-mocytoma, and acromegaly. These are not routinely screened for in hypertensive diabetic patients, and further investigation should be prompted by the presence of other clinical features.

4.1.1 **Investigation of hypertension in diabetic patients**

The measurement of blood pressure is an integral part of diabe-tes care, and in some clinical areas is measured at each visit. Blood pressure should be measured following the recommendations of the British Hypertension Society (Box 4.2). Hypertension in diabetes can be defined as a systolic blood pressure of 140 mmHg or over, and/or a diastolic blood pressure of 90 mmHg or over.

Ambulatory blood pressure monitoring (ABPM) or home blood pressure readings are usually lower than clinic readings, and thresh-olds and targets should be adjusted downwards by 10/5 mmHg. They are useful for identifying 'white coat' hypertension and for monitoring the response to treatment.

A diabetic patient with hypertension should have urea and elec-trolytes checked, with urinalysis for microalbuminuria and proteinuria. An ECG should be performed looking for voltage criteria of left ventricular hypertrophy. If present this carries a worse prognosis,

> **Box 4.2 British Hypertension Society recommendations for the measurement of blood pressure by standard mercury sphygmomanometer or semi-automated device**
>
> - Use a properly maintained, calibrated, and validated device
> - Measure sitting blood pressure routinely: standing blood pressures should be recorded if there is a suspicion of orthostatic hypotension
> - Remove tight clothing, support arm at heart level, ensure hand relaxed, and avoid talking during the measurement procedure
> - Use cuff of appropriate size
> - Lower mercury column slowly (2 mm/s)
> - Read blood pressure to the nearest 2 mmHg
> - Measure diastolic as disappearance of sounds (phase V)
> - Take the mean of at least two readings; more recordings are needed if notable differences between initial measurements are found
> - Do not treat on the basis of an isolated reading

and may influence the choice of antihypertensive drug. Imaging of the kidneys should be performed looking for renal artery stenosis if hypertension proves resistant to treatment.

4.2 Evidence of benefit in reducing blood pressure in diabetes

Patients with diabetes were excluded from many early trials of blood pressure lowering.

4.2.1 Studies in isolated systolic hypertension

The first clear evidence that blood pressure lowering was of benefit in people with diabetes was from studies in older patients with isolated systolic hypertension. As the study group was older, many subjects with diabetes were recruited, allowing diabetic sub-group analysis. The Systolic Hypertension in the Elderly Program (SHEP) study examined the use of clortalidone compared to placebo in systolic hypertension. There was a significant reduction in major cardiovascular events, with a greater absolute risk reduction in the diabetic subgroup. In the Systolic hypertension-Europe (Syst-Eur) study the benefits of nitrendipine compared with placebo were greater in the diabetic subgroup, with significant reductions in cardiovascular events, cardiovascular mortality, and all-cause mortality.

Together these studies demonstrated a significant reduction in cardiovascular events when hypertension was treated in people with diabetes.

4.2.2 **United Kingdom Prospective Diabetes Study**

The United Kingdom Prospective Diabetes Study (UKPDS), described in Chapter 2, and was a study of tight blood glucose control in patients with type 2 diabetes. During recruitment to the UKPDS the high prevalence of hypertension was noted, so a blood pressure study was nested within the main study, comparing tight blood pressure control (mean blood pressure 144/82 mmHg) with less tight control (mean 154/87 mmHg). One quarter of the total study population was also in the blood pressure study, and this was initially called the Hypertension in Diabetes Study (HDS). Tight control was obtained with a blood-pressure lowering regimen based on either captopril or atenolol, but many patients required three or more drugs.

Compared to the group with less tight control, tight control of blood pressure control reduced both macrovascular and microvascular complications of diabetes (Figure 4.1). No differences were observed comparing treatment based on captopril, with treatment based on atenolol, but the study was statistically underpowered for this comparison.

When the UKPDS patients were followed in post trial monitoring differences in blood pressure between the tight control and less tight control groups disappeared within two years of the termination of the trial. The significant reductions in vascular events were not maintained, indicating that good blood pressure control must be continued if the benefits are to be maintained, and there was no 'legacy' effect.

4.2.3 **Blood pressure targets in diabetes**

The Hypertension Optimal Treatment trial (HOT) was a larger but shorter study in 18,790 patients. The aim of the study was to compared the benefits of three diastolic blood pressure targets, <90 mmHg, <85 mmHg, and <80 mmHg, on major cardiovascular events (non-fatal myocardial infarction, non-fatal stroke, cardiovascular death). The separation between the groups was less than intended, and the achieved blood pressures were 144/85 mmHg, 141/83 mmHg and 140/81 mmHg.

In the study overall there was a reduction in major cardiovascular events comparing the group with a target blood pressure of <85 mmHg compared to a target of <90 mmHg, but there was no further benefit with a lower target of <80 mmHg. Post-hoc subgroup analysis of the 1,501 diabetic subjects (8%) showed a further significant reduction in major cardiovascular events in diabetic patients allocated to the lower target blood pressure.

The ADVANCE trial included a blood pressure lowering study comparing a fixed combination of perindopril plus indapamide with placebo and demonstrated that blood pressure lowering to even

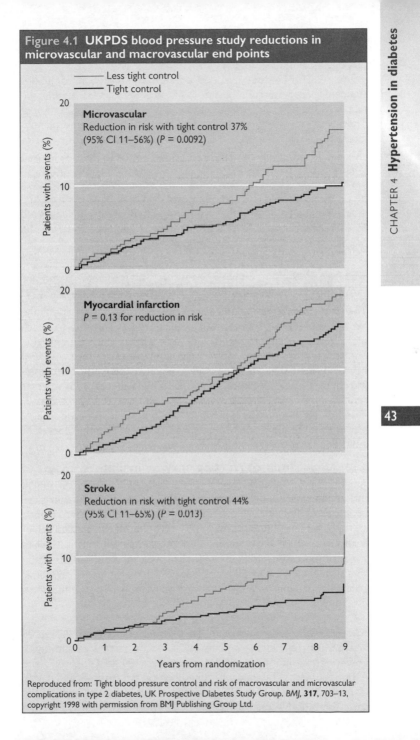

Figure 4.1 **UKPDS** blood pressure study reductions in microvascular and macrovascular end points

Less tight control
Tight control

Microvascular
Reduction in risk with tight control 37% (95% CI 11–56%) (P = 0.0092)

Myocardial infarction
P = 0.13 for reduction in risk

Stroke
Reduction in risk with tight control 44% (95% CI 11–65%) (P = 0.013)

Years from randomization

Reproduced from: Tight blood pressure control and risk of macrovascular and microvascular complications in type 2 diabetes, UK Prospective Diabetes Study Group. *BMJ*, **317**, 703–13, copyright 1998 with permission from BMJ Publishing Group Ltd.

lower levels (135/75 mmHg), and in patients not deemed to have hypertension at baseline, further reduced cardiovascular events in diabetic patients (Figure 4.2).

The ACCORD study included a blood pressure arm comparing standard therapy, targeting a systolic blood pressure <140 mmHg, and intensive therapy, targeting a systolic blood pressure <120 mmHg. There was no effect on the primary composite outcome of non-fatal myocardial infarction, nonfatal stroke or death from cardio-vascular causes. A slight significant reduction was seen in strokes (Figure 4.3).

When taken together these studies indicate that tight control of blood pressure reduces events more than less tight control, and indicate that a target blood pressure of <130/80 mmHg is supported by evidence, but that several agents may be required to reach the target.

4.3 **Which anti-hypertensive drug to use?**

The major benefit is the amount of blood pressure reduction, and many people with diabetes will require multiple agents to reach blood pressure targets, so the question is not 'which drug to use' but 'which drugs to use, and in what combinations?' Recent studies have indicated that atenolol is less effective than other therapies in reducing blood pressure in people with diabetes, with a lesser reduction in cardiovascular events, and first-line therapy is usually based on either an ACE inhibitor or angiotensin-II receptor antago-nist, with subsequent addition of either a calcium-channel blocker or a diuretic (Figure 4.4).

4.3.1 **Angiotensin-converting enzyme inhibitors**

Angiotensin-converting enzyme inhibitors (ACE inhibitors) inhibit the conversion of angiotensin I to angiotensin II. The main side-effects of ACE inhibitors are cough, hypotension, renal impairment, and angioedema. Cough is caused by inhibition of the breakdown of bradykinin, which by improving endothelial function might mediate some of the cardiovascular benefits of ACE inhibitors. ACE inhibi-tors slightly increase insulin sensitivity which may improve glycaemic control in patients with diabetes, and provoke hypoglycaemia when used in combination with oral antidiabetic drugs or insulin.

Captopril was demonstrated to reduce microvascular and mac-rovascular outcomes in the UKPDS blood pressure study. Lisinopril was one of the treatment arms in the Antihypertensive and Lipid-Lowering treatment to prevent Heart Attack Trial (ALLHAT) and perindopril was combined with amlodipine in the Anglo-Scandinavian Cardiac Outcomes (ASCOT) trial. Perindopril was also used as the basis for blood pressure treatment in the Perindopril Protection

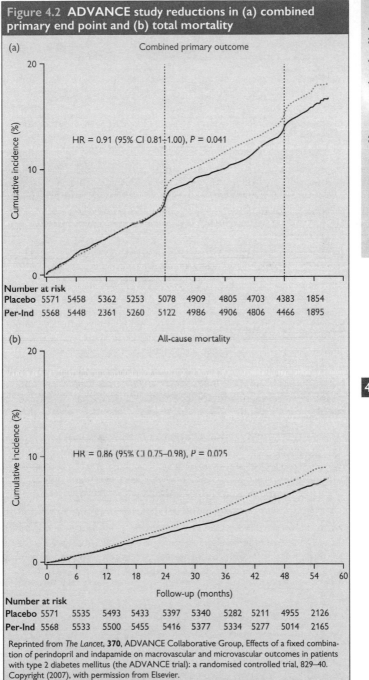

Figure 4.2 **ADVANCE** study reductions in (a) combined primary end point and (b) total mortality

(a) Combined primary outcome

Cumulative incidence (%)

HR = 0.91 (95% CI 0.81–1.00), *P* = 0.041

Number at risk
Placebo 5571 5458 5362 5253 5078 4909 4805 4703 4383 1854
Per-Ind 5568 5448 2361 5260 5122 4986 4906 4806 4466 1895

(b) All-cause mortality

Cumulative incidence (%)

HR = 0.86 (95% CI 0.75–0.98), *P* = 0.025

Follow-up (months)

Number at risk
Placebo 5571 5535 5493 5433 5397 5340 5282 5211 4955 2126
Per-Ind 5568 5533 5500 5455 5416 5377 5334 5277 5014 2165

Reprinted from *The Lancet*, **370**, ADVANCE Collaborative Group, Effects of a fixed combination of perindopril and indapamide on macrovascular and microvascular outcomes in patients with type 2 diabetes mellitus (the ADVANCE trial): a randomised controlled trial, 829–40. Copyright (2007), with permission from Elsevier.

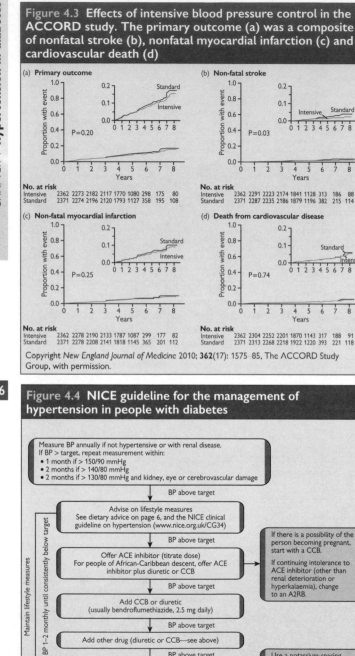

against Recurrent Stroke Study (PROGRESS) that is described in more detail in Chapter 9.

The ADVANCE study examined the use of a fixed dose combination of perindopril and indapamide compared to placebo in 11 140 patients with type 2 diabetes and cardiovascular disease or cardiovascular risk factors.

The potential benefits of ACE inhibitors on renal and cardiac outcomes in patients with diabetic nephropathy are described in Chapter 10.

4.3.2 Angiotensin-II receptor antagonists

Angiotensin-II receptor antagonists (ARAs) act highly selectively at angiotensin 1 (AT_1) receptors. Unlike ACE inhibitors, ARAs do not inhibit the breakdown of bradykinin, so are a useful alternative for patients that are unable to tolerate ACE inhibitors because of cough.

Losartan Intervention For Endpoint reduction in hypertension (LIFE) was a trial comparing losartan and atenolol-based therapy in 9,193 patients with hypertension and ECG criteria of left ventricular hypertrophy. Losartan significantly reduced the primary composite endpoint of cardiovascular death, myocardial infarction, and stroke, with significant reductions in stroke, but not myocardial infarction or cardiovascular death. In 1,195 patients with pre-existing diabetes (13%) losartan significantly reduced the composite endpoint, and cardiovascular and total mortality, but the reduction in strokes and myocardial infarction was not significant.

There have been several other publications from the LIFE study that have given useful information about cardiovascular risk in type 2 diabetes (Box 4.3).

The potential benefits of ARAs on renal and cardiac outcomes in patients with diabetic nephropathy are described in Chapter 10.

4.3.3 Calcium-channel blockers

Calcium-channel blockers were one of the first classes of drugs to be of proven benefit when used to treat hypertension in diabetes. Nitrendipine was used in the Syst-Eur study, and treatment in the HOT trial was based on felodipine. Initial concerns that nifedipine might increase myocardial infarctions in people with diabetes have not been substantiated.

Amlodipine was used in ALLHAT, ASCOT, and more recently in the Avoiding Cardiovascular Events through Combination Therapy in Patients Living with Systolic Hypertension (ACCOMPLISH) trial a combination of benazapril plus amlodipine was more effective at reducing cardiovascular events than a combination of benazapril plus hydrochlorothiazide. 60% of the participants had diabetes, and the reduction in cardiovascular events was slightly greater in diabetic than non-diabetic subjects.

Box 4.3 Results from the LIFE study
Principal result
• Losartan was more effective than atenolol in reducing the composite of cardiovascular death, myocardial infarction and stroke in hypertensive diabetic patients with ECG criteria of left ventricular hypertrophy
Other important results
• Losartan was more effective than atenolol in reducing sudden cardiac in people with diabetes
• Systolic and diastolic left ventricular function was impaired independent of left ventricular mass, most likely reflecting the adverse effects of diabetes on ventricular function
• Patients with diabetes had less regression of left ventricular hypertrophy in response to antihypertensive therapy than patients without diabetes
• Increasing baseline albuminuria related to increased risk for cardiovascular events in patients with diabetes, and benefits of losartan seemed to be greatest in patients with the highest baseline urinary albumin excretion
• The development of new-onset diabetes (NOD) could be predicted using a score based on baseline serum glucose concentration, body mass index, serum HDL cholesterol, systolic blood pressure and a history of prior use of antihypertensive drugs.

4.3.4 **Diuretics**

Bendroflumethiazide, formerly bendrofluazide, is a thiazide diuretic that is frequently recommended in treatment guidelines, but the evidence for its use in people with diabetes is remarkably slim. It was used in combination with atenolol in the ASCOT study.

Chlortalidone, formerly chlorthalidone, is a thiazide–related compound that reduced events in diabetic patients with systolic hypertension in the SHEP study. It was one of the treatment arms in the ALLHAT study which compared chlortalidone with lisinopril, amlodipine, and doxazosin. Lisinopril, amlodipine, and chlortalidone were equally effective, but this trial has been strongly criticised because of poor study design.

Indapamide is chemically related to chlortalidone, and is claimed to lower blood pressure with less metabolic disturbance. It was used as an optional part of the treatment in the PROGRESS study, and in fixed combination with perindopril in the ADVANCE study. Indapamide was also used in the Hypertension in the Very Elderly Trial (HYVET) which demonstrated reduction in cardiovascular events by treating hypertension in people over 80 years of age. Few diabetic subjects were included.

4.3.5 Beta-blockers

Most of the evidence for the use of beta-blockers in diabetes concerns atenolol. In the UKPDS atenolol was as effective as the ACE-inhibitor captopril in reducing microvascular and macrovascular events, although in retrospect the study was underpowered to show any difference. In the LIFE study atenolol was inferior to losartan in reducing the primary composite endpoint of cardiovascular death, myocardial infarction and stroke.

More recently the ASCOT study compared newer treatments (amlodipine plus perindopril) versus older treatments (atenolol plus bendroflumethiazide) in 19257 patients with hypertension and cardiovascular risk. 5145 subjects (27%) were known to have diabetes at randomization.

The study was stopped early because of a significant reduction in total mortality comparing newer and older treatments. The reduction in the primary endpoint (non-fatal myocardial infarction, cardiovascular death) was not statistically significant, but most of the secondary endpoints were significantly reduced.

The study was designed to give equal effectiveness in reducing blood pressure, but in fact the newer treatments were more effect, with a mean blood pressure of 136/78 mmHg with newer treatments versus 138/79 for older treatments. When a statistical correction was made for the difference in blood pressures, the newer treatments were still more effective in reducing vascular endpoints.

Because of the results of ASCOT and LIFE beta-blockers are no longer recommended as first-line antihypertensive drugs unless there is another indication for their use such as post-myocardial infarction, chronic heart failure, or the symptomatic treatment of angina.

4.3.6 Other agents

Doxazosin is an alpha-blocker. The doxazosin arm of ALLHAT was stopped prematurely, and doxazosin should be reserved for diabetic patients that are unable to tolerate alternatives or have not reached blood pressure targets despite multiple drugs.

4.4 Risks of diabetes with anti-hypertensive drugs

The development of new-onset diabetes (NOD) has been a secondary endpoint in several blood pressure and cardiovascular trials. Beta-blockers and diuretics increase the risk of new-onset diabetes, and calcium-channel blockers are neutral. ACE-inhibitors and ARAs

Box 4.4 Possible explanations for the reduction in new-onset diabetes with ACE inhibitors and ARAs

Blockade of adverse effects of angiotensin II

- Improved insulin signalling
- Improved skeletal muscle blood flow
- Reduced oxidative stress
- Reduced sympathetic activation
- Suppressed adipogenesis
- Increased islet cell blood flow

Effects beyond the renin-angiotensin system

- Enhanced glucose metabolism by activation of bradykinin/nitric oxide pathways (ACE inhibitors)
- Improved glucose and lipid metabolism by activation of PPAR gamma

seem to reduce the development of NOD in cardiovascular patients and there are several hypothetical explanations for this (Box 4.4). In the Nateglinide and Valsartan in Impaired Glucose Tolerance Outcomes Research (NAVIGATOR) study valsartan slightly, but significantly, reduced the progression to diabetes, but had no effect on cardiovascular outcomes. In the Diabetes REduction Assessment with ramipril and rosiglitazone Medication (DREAM) trial ramipril treatment did not significantly effect the progression to diabetes. Regression to normoglycaemia, which was a secondary endpoint, was significantly increased with ramipril.

4.5 **Conclusions**

The management of hypertension in patients with diabetes has been proven to reduce macrovascular and microvascular endpoints. Several drug classes are of proven benefit, and multiple drugs may be required to reach blood pressure targets.

References

The ACCORD Study Group (2010) Effects of intensive blood pressure control in type 2 diabetes. *New England Journal of Medicine* **362**: 1575–85.

ADVANCE Collaborative Group (2007) Effects of a fixed combination of perindopril and indapamide on macrovascular and microvascular outcomes in patients with type 2 diabetes mellitus (the ADVANCE trial): a randomised controlled trial. *Lancet* **370**: 829–40.

ALLHAT Officers and Coordinators for the ALLHAT Collaborative Research Group (2002) Major outcomes in high-risk hypertensive patients randomized to angiotensin-converting enzyme inhibitor or calcium channel blocker vs diuretic: The Antihypertensive and Lipid-Lowering Treatment to Prevent Heart Attack Trial (ALLHAT). *Journal of the American Medical Association* **288**: 2981–97.

Curb JD, Pressel SL, Cutler JA, et al. (1996) Effect of diuretic-based anti-hypertensive treatment on cardiovascular disease risk in older diabetic patients with isolated systolic hypertension. *Journal of the American Medical Association* **276**: 1886–92.

Dahlof B, Sever PS, Poulter NR, et al., for the ASCOT investigators (2005) Prevention of cardiovascular events with an antihypertensive regimen of amlodipine adding perindopril as required versus atenolol adding bendro-flumethiazide as required, in the Anglo-Scandinavian Cardiac Outcomes Trial-Blood Pressure Lowering Arm (ASCOT-BPLA): a multicentre randomised controlled trail. *Lancet* **366**: 895–906.

Hansson L, Zanchetti A, Carruthers SG, et al., for the HOT Study Group (1998) Effects of intensive blood-pressure lowering and low-dose aspirin in patients with hypertension: principal results of the Hypertension Optimal Treatment (HOT) randomised trial. *Lancet* **351**: 1755–62.

Holman RR, Paul SK, Bethel MA, Neil HAW, Mathews DR (2008) Long-term follow-up after tight control of blood pressure in type 2 diabetes. *New England Journal of Medicine* **359**: 1565–76.

Lindholm LH, Ibsen H, Dahlöf B, et al., for the LIFE study group (2002) Cardiovascular morbidity and mortality in patients with diabetes in the Losartan Intervention For Endpoint reduction in hypertension study (LIFE): a randomised trial against atenolol. *Lancet* **359**: 1004–10.

Tuomilehto J, Rastenyte D, Birkenhager WH, et al., for the Systolic Hypertension in Europe Trial Investigators (1999). Effects of calcium-channel blockade in older patients with diabetes and systolic hypertension. *New England Journal of Medicine* **340**: 677–84.

UK Prospective Diabetes Study Group (1998) Tight blood pressure control and risk of macrovascular and microvascular complications in type 2 diabetes: UKPDS 38. *British Medical Journal* **317**: 703–13.

Weber MA, Bakris GL, Jamerson K et al., for the ACCOMPLISH Investigators (2010) Cardiovascular events during differing hypertnsion therapies in patients with diabetes. *Journal of the American College of Cardiology* **56**: 77–85.

Chapter 5

Coronary heart disease in diabetes

Adil Rajwani and Stephen Wheatcroft

Key points

- Cardiovascular disease is the commonest cause of death in individuals with diabetes
- The presence of diabetes may be regarded as a 'cardiovascular disease equivalent', conferring the same risk of future cardiovascular events as the presence of established cardiovascular disease
- Hyperglycaemia, insulin resistance, oxidative stress, dyslipidaemia, inflammation, and clotting abnormalities are all implicated in increased atherothrombosis in diabetes
- Individuals with diabetes have more severe and rapidly progressive coronary artery disease, with greater multi-vessel and left main coronary artery involvement
- The proportion of individuals with non typical symptoms or silent ischaemia is increased in the presence of diabetes
- Whether asymptomatic individuals with diabetes should be screened for the presence of cardiovascular disease remains unclear at present
- Intensive secondary prevention is essential with anti-platelet, anti-hypertensive and lipid-lowering treatment.

53

5.1 Background

5.1.1 Epidemiology

Cardiovascular diseases account for up to 75% of all deaths in patients with diabetes. The risk of death from coronary heart disease (CHD) in individuals with diabetes is two- to three-fold greater than in those without diabetes. Women with diabetes are particularly prone to cardiovascular disease. The increased cardiovascular risk attributable to diabetes is only partly explained by concomitant risk factors including hypertension, obesity, dyslipidaemia, and smoking. This suggests that components of the diabetes phenotype, including hyperglycaemia, insulin resistance, inflammation, endothelial dysfunction, and oxidative stress, are important mediators of the elevated CHD risk and increased mortality.

Although age-adjusted mortality rates for cardiovascular disease in the general population have been declining recent years, there has been an increase in mortality in patients with diabetes.

A large prospective study in a Finnish population demonstrated that patients with type 2 diabetes but without prior myocardial infarction (MI) had a risk of MI during follow-up that was similar to that of non-diabetic patients who had already had a prior MI. Although subsequent studies have not corroborated these findings in other populations, this study prompted the recommendation that diabetes should be regarded as a 'cardiovascular disease equivalent' when estimating cardiovascular risk.

5.2 **Pathology**

5.2.1 **Plaque development**

Atherosclerotic plaques develop through a complex process resulting from endothelial cell dysfunction, adhesion and incorporation of inflammatory cells, lipid deposition, smooth muscle cell proliferation, and changes in intercellular matrix. The factors which may contribute to atherosclerosis in diabetes are illustrated in Figure 5.1.

Endothelial cell dysfunction, one of the earliest detectable vascular abnormalities in individuals who subsequently develop atherosclerosis, is a key factor in plaque development and progression. Characterized by an imbalance in the production of pro- and anti-atherosclerotic molecules by endothelial cells, endothelial dysfunction is closely related to insulin resistance and may precede the development of type 2 diabetes by many years. In fact, insulin resistance has emerged as a unifying aetiologic factor linking type 2 diabetes with atherosclerosis.

Hyperglycaemia contributes to atherosclerosis by multiple mechanisms, including increased production of advanced glycation end products (AGE), which favour overproduction of reactive oxygen species. Increased expression of adhesion molecules by endothelial cells and production of pro-inflammatory chemokines and cytokines promote infiltration of macrophages and other inflammatory cells. Diabetes favours uptake of oxidized LDL and stimulates

Figure 5.1 Diabetes is associated with multiple abnormalities which induce endothelial dysfunction. This shifts the balance between the production of molecules such as nitric oxide (NO) and endothelin (ET)-1, favouring the development of atherosclerosis

macrophages to form lipid-laden foam cells. Diabetes is also associated with vascular smooth muscle cell proliferation. Apoptosis of inflammatory cells and smooth muscle cells contributes to the formation of the necrotic core. Increased expression of matrix metalloproteinases in diabetes permits plaque remodelling and may favour plaque rupture.

Post-mortem studies comparing hearts from individuals with and without diabetes who have died suddenly confirm a greater total plaque load, with a predisposition to distal coronary artery location and larger necrotic cores, in individuals with diabetes. Plaques from patients with diabetes have greater numbers of macrophages and T-lymphocytes, increased expression of receptors for advanced glycation end products and more smooth muscle cell and macrophage apoptosis.

5.2.2 **Vessel remodelling**
In the early stages of plaque development, the coronary artery typically remodels outward, thereby maintaining a near-normal lumen.

In individuals with diabetes, however, both pathological and intra-vascular ultrasound studies demonstrate that the vessel remodels inward. This results in significant luminal compromise by the developing plaque, promoting ischaemic symptoms and favouring coronary occlusion subsequent to plaque rupture.

5.2.3 **Hypercoagulability**

Clinical manifestations of plaque rupture are attributable to the formation of a platelet-rich thrombus. Diabetes is associated with a number of abnormalities promoting platelet aggregation and thrombus formation. Platelets are larger in individuals with diabetes, with greater expression of glycoprotein IIb/IIa and increased tendency to aggregate compared to individuals without diabetes. Circulating concentrations of coagulation factors VII, XII and fibrinogen are increased, as are plasma levels of the fibrinolytic inhibitor, plasminogen activator inhibitor-1. In addition, diabetes has important effects on fibrin structure and function, generating a clot with a denser structure which is more resistant to lysis.

5.3 **Features of coronary disease in diabetes**

5.3.1 **Pathological studies**

Large autopsy studies have demonstrated that severity and extent of coronary artery disease are markedly increased in patients with diabetes. In a recent population-based post-mortem study, high grade coronary stenoses were found in 75% of men and women with diabetes, in contrast to 55% of those without diabetes. After adjusting for age and sex, the likelihood of a high atherosclerosis burden was equivalent in patients with diabetes without clinical coronary heart diease and in patients without diabetes with clinical coronary heart disease. The study revealed high prevalence of sub-clinical coronary artery disease in individuals with diabetes without a history of coronary heart disease.

Debulking of atherosclerotic plaques by percutaneous coronary intervention with directional coronary atherectomy allows the plaque debris to be exported and examined histologically. Plaque debris from patients with diabetes has a significantly higher macrophage contact than that from individuals without diabetes.

5.3.2 **Angiographic studies**

Angiographic series confirm a greater atherosclerotic burden in patients with diabetes. A recent single-centre study compared the findings of consecutive patients undergoing coronary angiography according to the presence or absence of diabetes. Coronary disease, evaluated objectively with a severity scoring system, was more severe in the patients with diabetes and included higher coronary occlusion rates. In other angiographic studies the presence of diabetes was associated with more diffuse, multi-vessel, left main, and distal coronary artery disease with poorer collateral development.

5.3.3 Intra-vascular ultrasound studies

Intra-vascular ultrasound allows detailed information on vessel wall and plaque morphology to be gathered at the time of coronary angiography. Diabetes is a strong independent predictor of atheroma volume assessed using this technique. Virtual histology, in which plaque composition is inferred from spectral analysis of ultrasound reflected from the plaque, reveals that diabetes is associated with more plaque calcification, larger necrotic cores and a greater prevalence of rupture prone thin cap fibro-atheroma.

5.4 Investigation

5.4.1 Choice of investigation

Investigation may be carried out to confirm the presence of CHD in patients with suggestive symptoms or to screen for CHD in asymptomatic individuals. Choice of modality is influenced by patient-specific factors, in particular the ability to exercise, and by local availability. Functional imaging (nuclear imaging, stress echocardiography and stress magnetic resonance imaging) detect coronary artery disease indirectly by assessing myocardial ischaemia induced by coronary stenoses, whereas X-ray angiography affords direct visualization of the coronary arteries. Other techniques, such as coronary calcium scoring, are less useful in the diagnosis of coronary artery disease but may have a role in screening and risk stratification.

5.4.2 Exercise electrocardiography

Exercise electrocardiography (ECG) is widely used but has a lower diagnostic accuracy than perfusion imaging. An adverse prognosis is indicated by poor exercise capacity, exercise-induced ST-segment depression, chronotropic incompetence, or a fall in systolic blood pressure. Sensitivity of exercise ECG is reduced if the patient is unable to achieve 85% of maximal predicted heart rate response to stress. Up to half of patients with diabetes may be unable to achieve this. Other limitations of exercise electrocardiography include respiratory, neurological or orthopaedic conditions which preclude exercise and resting ECG abnormalities (e.g. left bundle branch block, left ventricular hypertrophy, ventricular pacing, or digoxin use) which prevent interpretation of ST segment changes with stress.

5.4.3 **Nuclear myocardial perfusion imaging**

The diagnostic utility of single-photon emission computed tomography (SPECT) imaging with pharmacological stress has been extensively demonstrated in the general population, although studies in specifically in individuals with diabetes are scarce. The presence of perfusion abnormalities is strongly predictive of subsequent cardiac death and non-fatal myocardial infarction in both symptomatic and asymptomatic populations with diabetes. Clinical outcomes are directly related to the severity and size of the perfusion abnormalities. A 'normal' SPECT scan has a lower negative predictive value for future cardiovascular events in patients with diabetes than in the general population. This may reflect the more rapid progression of atherosclerosis in patients with diabetes.

5.4.4 **Stress echocardiography**

Stress echocardiography assesses regional myocardial wall motion in response to exercise or, more usually, pharmacological stress. In unselected populations, stress echocardiography has similar sensitivity and specificity for detection of coronary artery disease to SPECT imaging. Small scale studies in individuals with diabetes support a similar sensitivity and specificity to non-diabetic individuals. Several studies have confirmed that stress-induced wall motion abnormalities predict cardiovascular death and non-fatal myocardial infarction in patients with diabetes. Similar to the SPECT imaging, the severity of echocardiographic abnormalities predict long-term prognosis and the negative-predictive value of stress echocardiography is diminished in individuals with diabetes.

5.4.5 **Cardiac magnetic resonance imaging**

Cardiac magnetic resonance imaging (MRI) allows comprehensive assessment of myocardial perfusion, viability, coronary anatomy, and global and regional ventricular function in a single study. The high spatial resolution of MRI allows even small perfusion defects to be detected and permits differentiation between subendocardial and transmural infarction. Senstivity and specificity of cardiac MRI for detection of coronary artery disease in the general population are high but specific studies in patients with diabetes are not available.

5.4.6 **Coronary artery calcium scoring**

Electron-beam computed tomography (EBCT) and multi-slice computed tomography (MSCT) allow non-invasive detection and quantification of coronary artery calcification. Coronary calcium scores are closely correlated with total atherosclerotic burden and the risk of future cardiovascular events, but do not predict the severity of coronary stenoses or provide anatomical information. In the general population, the coronary calcium score may provide incremental prognostic information over conventional risk stratification, particularly in individuals at 'intermediate' risk. Limited data are available on coronary artery calcium scoring in individuals with diabetes, although recent studies support the calcium score as an important predictor of mortality, with a greater increase in mortality rate attributable to incremental increases in calcium score in subjects with diabetes that in those without.

5.4.7 X-ray coronary angiography

Coronary angiography remains the definitive investigation for the evaluation of coronary artery disease and provides anatomical information on the extent and distribution of disease which is essential for planning subsequent revascularization. There is a small, but not insignificant, incidence of severe complications (death, myocardial infarction or stroke), at approximately 0.1–0.2%. The occurrence of contrast-induced nephropathy is significantly greater in individuals with diabetes (particularly in pre existing renal impairment) and meticulous attention to pre-hydration should be made wherever possible.

5.4.8 Non-invasive coronary angiography

Recent technical developments in cardiac MRI and MSCT have allowed both techniques to be proposed as alternatives to X-ray angiography. The high spatial resolution and fast scan times of MSCT are particularly attractive for non-invasive angiography. In the general population, the high sensitivity and specificity of MSCT to detect coronary artery disease has led to increasing uptake of this technique. Validation studies of MSCT in patients with diabetes reveal more diseased coronary segments and more frequent obstructive disease in comparison to patients without diabetes.

5.5 Presentation

5.5.1 Symptoms of coronary heart disease

CHD frequently presents without typical symptoms in individuals with diabetes. The prevalence of 'silent ischaemia' is much higher in those with diabetes than in the general population. Almost one-third of myocardial infarctions in patients with diabetes are not accompanied by chest pain. This may reflect underlying autonomic dysfunction or differences in pain sensitivity associated with diabetes. Similarly, easy fatigability, atypical thoracic discomfort or effort-related dyspnoea may be the only indications of stable coronary artery disease in patients with diabetes.

5.5.2 Silent ischaemia

The true prevalence of coronary artery disease in asymptomatic individuals with diabetes is not known. Estimates vary between studies, depending on the imaging modality, study selection criteria and background risk of the population. The prevalence of coronary atherosclerosis, evaluated using EBCT-derived calcium score, was 46.3% in a study of over 500 asymptomatic patients with diabetes. Several studies have evaluated silent ischemia, using nuclear imaging or stress echocardiography.

In the Detection of Silent Myocardial Ischaemic in Asymptomatic Diabetics (DIAD) study, the prevalence of abnormal SPECT scans in 522 asymptomatic patients with diabetes and two or more risk factors was 21%. Conventional risk factors did not predict perfusion defects on SPECT. Other studies using SPECT or stress echocardiography suggest a higher prevalence of silent ischaemia (see Table 5.1). All studies in which subsequent clinical events were evaluated confirm a substantially higher risk of cardiovascular death or myocardial infarction in patients with evidence of atherosclerosis or silent ischaemia.

5.6 **Screening**

The high prevalence of atherosclerosis and silent ischaemia has prompted some authors and organizations to recommend screening for coronary artery disease in asymptomatic individuals with diabetes. However, this approach is controversial and is not supported by the current evidence base. Studies using SPECT imaging or stress echocardiography suggest that selecting patients with diabetes for screening on the basis of established risk factors would fail to identify a large proportion of individuals with asymptomatic coronary artery disease. Additionally, although it is likely that high-risk asymptomatic individuals identified by screening would be targeted for intensive medical therapy, there is a lack of evidence that revascularization improves clinical outcomes. In the large Bypass Angioplasty

Table 5.1 **Prevalence of atherosclerosis or silent ischaemia in asymptomatic individuals with diabetes**

Study (year of publication)	Participants	Modality	Prevalence of abnormal study
Anand et al (2006)	510	EBCT	46.3%
Sconamiglio et al (2006)	1899	Stress Echo	60%
Wackers et al (2004)	522	SPECT	21%
Miller et al (2004)	1738	SPECT	59%
Zellweger et al (2004)	1737	SPECT	39%
Rajagopalan et al (2005)	1427	SPECT	58%

Revascularization Investigation 2 Diabetes (BARI 2-D) study, there was no difference in rates of death and major cardiovascular events between patients randomized to prompt revascularization compared to those randomized to medical therapy. A pragmatic approach, therefore, is to treat established diabetes as a 'cardiovascular risk equivalent' and target all individuals with diabetes with intensive medical therapy and lifestyle advice. A recent consensus statement from the American Diabetes Association suggests that screening, perhaps with cardiac CT, should be reserved for those in whom medical treatment goals cannot be met and in individuals in whom there is strong clinical suspicion of very high-risk coronary artery disease.

5.7 Symptomatic treatment

Anti-anginal therapy improves symptoms by redressing the imbalance between myocardial perfusion and oxygen demand.

5.7.1 Beta-blockers

These improve symptom frequency and severity by reducing myocardial oxygen demand. Slowing of resting and exercise-induced heart rate is important in their mode of action. Beta-blockers are effective anti-anginal agents which are generally recommended as first-line therapy in patients with or without diabetes.

5.7.2 Nitrates

Nitrates are vasodilators which increase subendocardial perfusion by reducing preload (and thus LV end-diastolic pressures and wall-stress) and promoting coronary and collateral dilatation. A nitrate-free period is required with long-acting agents to avoid tolerance. Short-acting sub-lingual or buccal nitrates provide rapid symptom relief and can be used prophylactically.

5.7.3 Calcium antagonists

Inhibition of calcium influx in vascular smooth muscle cells promotes relaxation, thereby increasing coronary blood flow and systemic vasodilatation. Diltiazem and verapamil have negative chronotropic properties and are useful alternatives to beta-blockers.

5.7.4 Other antianginal agents

Nicorandil has nitrate-like properties and also vasodilates by opening potassium channels. It is an effective anti-anginal and reduced the risk of cardiovascular events during follow-up in a randomised trial of patients with stable coronary artery disease. The protective effect was consistent in the sub-group with diabetes, although the trial excluded patients with diabetes who were receiving a suplphonylurea. Ivabradine, a selective I(f) channel blocker, improves anginal symptoms by limiting heart rate through direct effects on the sinus node. Ivabradine may be considered in beta-blocker intolerant individuals or in those in whom resting heart rate is not adequately controlled by a beta-blocker. Ranolazine is a novel anti-anginal, which reduces ichaemia by inhibiting the late phase of the inward sodium current, thereby reducing intracellular sodium and calcium overload. Ranolazine may have advantages in patients with diabetes, as it was demonstrated to reduce recurrent ischaemia and significantly improve HbA1c concentrations in a large trial in patients with acute coronary syndrome.

5.8 **Secondary prevention**

5.8.1 **Anti-platelets**

Aspirin is recommended in all patients with coronary artery disease, although it is recognized that its efficacy may be diminished in those with diabetes. In a recent large meta-analysis, treatment with aspirin conferred a 22% reduction in vascular events overall, whilst in the sub-group with diabetes, the 7% relative risk reduction did not reach statistical significance. A post-hoc analysis of the sub-group with diabetes in the Clopidogrel versus Aspirin in Patients at Risk of Ischemic Events (CAPRIE) study found that clopidogrel reduced the risk of death, myocardial infarction, stroke or hospital admission compared with aspirin in patients with a history of atherothrombosis. Anti-platelet therapy in acute coronary syndromes is discussed in Chapter 6.

5.8.2 **Beta-blockers**

Beta-blockers reduce mortality following myocardial infarction and improve symptoms and mortality in patients with heart failure. Beta-blockers are particularly effective in reducing post-infarction mortality in patients with diabetes and are recommended in all patients with coronary artery disease who have experienced an ischaemic event.

5.8.3 **Angiotensin converting enzyme inhibitors**

Angiotensin converting enzyme (ACE) inhibitors improve symptoms and mortality in patients with left ventricular systolic dysfunction and prior MI. The effect is consistent in patients with and without diabetes. ACE inhibitors also improve outcomes in patients with preserved left ventricular function, diabetes, and cardiovascular disease. Ramipril reduced cardiovascular events in patients with diabetes and a previous cardiovascular event or at least one risk factor in the Microalbuminuria, Cardiovascular and Renal Outcomes-Heart Outcomes Prevention Evaluation (MICRO-HOPE) substudy. A similar risk reduction was conferred by perinodopril in the diabetes sub-group of the EURopean trial On reduction of cardiac events with Perindopril in stable coronary Artery disease (EUROPA). In the Prevention of Events with Angiotensin Converting Enzyme inhibition (PEACE) study, however, trandolapril did not reduce the risk of cardiovascular events in patients with established coronary heart disease. This may reflect a lower risk study population and suboptimal dosing. Meta-analysis of available trials strongly supports the use of ACE inhibitors in all patients with diabetes and coronary heart disease.

5.8.4 Lipid-lowering agents

The appropriate use of lipid-lowering therapy in individuals with diabetes is discussed in Chapter 3.

5.9 Conclusions

Coronary heart disease is the commonest cause of death in patients with diabetes. Although individuals with diabetes and cardiovascular disease benefit from secondary preventive strategies to similar, if not greater, extent than their counterparts without diabetes, they remain at substantially higher absolute risk of morbidity and mortality. Further research is warranted to more fully understand and resolve this 'residual risk' attributable to diabetes.

References

BARI 2D Study Group; Frye RL, August P, Brooks MM, et al. (2009) A randomized trial of therapies for type 2 diabetes and coronary artery disease. New England Journal of Medicine **360**: 2503 15.

Bax JJ, Inzucchi SE, Bonow RO, Schuljf JD, Freeman MR, Barrett EJ (2007) Cardiac imaging for risk stratification in diabetes. Diabetes Care **30**: 1295–1304.

Bax JJ, Young LH, Frye RL, Bonow RO, Steinberg HO, Barrett EJ; ADA (2007) Screening for coronary artery disease in patients with diabetes. Diabetes Care **30**: 2729–36.

Fox K, Garcia MA, Ardissino D, et al. (2006) Guidelines on the management of stable angina pectoris: executive summary: the Task Force on the Management of Stable Angina Pectoris of the European Society of Cardiology. European Heart Journal **27**: 1341–81.

Haffner SM, Lehto S, Ronnemaa T, Pyorala K, Laakso M (1998) Mortality from coronary heart dieuse in subjects with type 2 diabetes and in nondiabetic sunjects with and without prior myocardial infarction. New England Journal of Medicine **339**: 229–34.

Heart Outcomes Prevention Evaluation Study Investigators (2000) Effects of ramipril on cardiovascular and microvascular outcomes in people with diabetes mellitus: results of the HOPE study and MICRO-HOPE substudy. *Lancet* **355**: 253–9.

Ryden L, Standl E, Bartnik M, Van den BG, Betteridge J, de Boer MJ (2007) Guidelines on diabetes, pre-diabetes, and cardiovascular diseases: executive summary. The Task Force on Diabetes and Cardiovascular Diseases of the European Society of Cardiology (ESC) and of the European Association for the Study of Diabetes (EASD). *European Heart Journal* **28**: 88–136.

Wackers FJ, Young LH, Inzucchi SE, *et al.* (2004) Detection of silent myocardial ischemia in asymptomatic diabetic subjects: the DIAD study. *Diabetes Care* **27**: 1954–61.

Chapter 6

Acute coronary syndromes in diabetes

Matthew Kahn and Stephen Wheatcroft

> **Key points**
>
> - Individuals with diabetes have an increased incidence of acute coronary syndromes (ACS) and experience poorer outcomes compared with those without diabetes
> - Despite data suggesting that patients with diabetes derive greater benefit from evidence-based therapies for ACS than those without diabetes, these patients less commonly receive treatment according to established guidelines (particularly insulin-treated patients)
> - Appropriate management of ACS in patients with diabetes mandates prompt treatment with anti-thrombotic and anti-ischaemic medication, early access to effective reperfusion and revascularization, and institution of optimal secondary preventive measures.

6.1 Clinical features

6.1.1 Epidemiology

The presence of diabetes is common in patients presenting with acute coronary syndromes (ACS). Around 20–25% of patients with ACS are reported to have diabetes in multi-national registries. In addition, a substantial proportion of patients with ACS who are not known to have diabetes have will have abnormalities when challenged with an oral glucose tolerance test. Overall, 65% of patients presenting with acute myocardial infarction have demonstrable evidence of impaired glucoregulation.

6.1.2 **Pathogenesis**

Acute coronary syndromes (ACS) arise as a consequence of an athero-thrombotic process, typically initiated by spontaneous rupture or erosion of an atherosclerotic coronary plaque. Exposure of the plaque constituents to circulating blood promotes platelet aggregation and thrombosis. Myocardial ischaemia results from thrombotic occlusion of the vessel, or from distal embolization of sub-occlusive thrombus compounded by vasospasm.

A number of factors predispose individuals with diabetes to plaque rupture, as illustrated in Figure 6.1. Insulin resistance, oxidative stress and hyperglycaemia are associated with endothelial dysfunction—a key feature in the development and progression of atherosclerosis.

The presence of diabetes is also linked with increased vascular inflammation, characterized by greater lymphocytic infiltration, increased production of pro-inflammatory cytokines and upregulation of matrix metalloproteinases which predispose the plaque to rupture. Diabetes is also associated with a pro-thrombotic state. Platelets are larger with an increased propensity to adhere to the vessel wall. A greater concentration of cell surface glycoprotein IIb/IIIa receptors facilitates aggregation upon stimulation. Altered clotting factors and reduced concentrations of endogenous fibrinolytic mediators in individuals with diabetes are complicit in increasing the likelihood of a plaque rupture resulting in thrombotic complications and the clinical manifestation of an ACS.

6.1.3 **Influence of diabetes on clinical outcomes**

Despite implementation of contemporary evidence based therapies, diabetes confers an adverse prognosis for patients presenting

Figure 6.1 Factors promoting atherosclerosis and plaque rupture in individuals with diabetes

Altered clotting factors

Inflammatory cell adhesion & incorporation

Plaque rupture

Increased platelet activation & aggregation

Endothelial cell dysfunction

Increased cytokine production

Increased matrix metalloproteinase activity

with ACS. Both short-term outcomes and long-term survival are substantially impaired in individuals with diabetes following ACS.

Diabetes increases the risk of a range of complications following ACS, including left ventricular dysfunction, symptomatic heart failure, recurrent myocardial ischaemia, requirement for urgent revascularization, cardiogenic shock, arrythmias, re-infarction, stroke, and death. The risk of adverse events is greater in insulin-treated patients with diabetes than in those treated with oral hypoglycaemic agents or diet alone.

In the large multi-national 'Global Registry of Acute Coronary Events' (GRACE), which assessed outcomes in over 16,000 patients with ACS, approximately one in four patients studied had diabetes. The patients with diabetes were less likely to receive effective therapies and were at increased risk of heart failure, renal failure, cardiogenic shock, and death. These differences remained after adjustment for potentially confounding factors. Further observations from GRACE revealed that mortality at 30 days and one year was significantly higher amongst patients with diabetes than those without diabetes presenting with ACS.

6.1.4 Classification of ACS
Acute coronary syndromes, in individuals with compatible symptoms, are classified on the basis of the index electrocardiogram (see Table 6.1). ST-segment elevation usually signifies the presence of an occlusive thrombus and mandates emergency reperfusion (by mechanical or pharmacological means) in order to salvage the myocardium under jeopardy. Ischaemic symptoms without ST-segment elevation usually reflect sub-occlusive thrombus. Patients presenting in this manner are typically treated with intensive anti-thrombotic and anti-ischaemic medication, before being considered for urgent coronary angiography and revascularization, if appropriate, following risk stratification. Myocardial infarction is diagnosed on the basis of clinical symptoms, elevation of biomarkers of cardiomyocyte necrosis or electrocardiographic changes.

6.2 Non ST-segment elevation acute coronary syndromes

6.2.1 Antiplatelet therapy
Platelet activation and aggregation, which play a key role in mediating the clinical features of ACS following rupture of an atherosclerotic plaque, are exaggerated in the presence of diabetes. Intensive antiplatelet therapy is, therefore, a crucial component of the therapeutic approach to ACS.

Table 6.1 Classification and management of acute coronary syndromes

	ST-segment elevation (STE-ACS)	Non ST-segment elevation (NSTE-ACS)
Typical ECG changes	ST-segment elevation (or new left bundle-branch block)	ST-segment depression, T-wave inversion, may be normal
Typical pathology	Plaque rupture → occlusive thrombus	Plaque rupture → non-occlusive thrombus
Immediate management	Reperfusion to limit myocardial necrosis with primary percutaneous coronary intervention if available, or, fibrinolysis	Intensive medical therapy with anti-platelet, anti-thrombotic and anti-ischaemic agents
Early management	Monitoring on coronary care unit	Coronary angiography & revascularization if appropriate
Longer term management	Life-style measures, anti-platelet agents, beta-blockers, angiotensin converting enzyme inhibitors, lipid lowering therapy, cardiac rehabilitation programme.	

The benefit of aspirin in athero-thrombotic disease is well established. Although questions remain over the efficacy of aspirin in the primary prevention of cardiovascular disease in diabetes, its use in the acute setting remains universal.

The thienopyridine drugs (e.g. ticlopidine, clopidogrel, and prasugrel) and the novel non-thienopyridine drug ticagrelor inhibit platelet aggregation in a synergistic manner to aspirin by blocking adenosine diphosphate receptor–dependent platelet activation through inhibition of the P2Y12 receptor. The pivotal 'Clopidogrel in Unstable Angina to Prevent Recurrent Events' (CURE) study examined whether the addition of clopidogrel to aspirin in the context of non ST-segment elevation ACS improved outcome. The addition of clopidogrel to aspirin resulted in a 20% reduction in the composite endpoint of cardiovascular death, myocardial infarction or stroke after 12 months of follow-up. The 2,840 participants with diabetes had a higher overall vascular event rate than their counterparts without diabetes. The event rate was reduced to a similar extent by the addition of clopidogrel in this group, although this did not reach statistical significance. Recently, two large randomized trials have compared the novel P2Y12 inhibitors prasugrel and ticagrelor with clopidogrel in patients with acute coronary syndromes. In the

TRITON-TIMI 38 study, prasugrel significantly reduced the composite endpoint of cardiovascular death, myocardial infarction and stroke compared to clopidogrel in 13,608 patients with acute coronary syndrome scheduled to undergo PCI, although at the expense of an increased the risk of bleeding. Interestingly, a pre-specified subgroup with diabetes receiving prasugrel in this trial had a greater reduction in ischaemic events without an increased risk of bleeding, indicating a net clinical benefit in patients with diabetes treated with prasugrel. In the PLATO study, ticagrelor significantly reduced the risk of cardiovascular death, myocardial infarction or stroke in 18,624 patients with acute coronary syndrome compared to clopidogrel, without an increase in major bleeding.

Platelets from individuals with diabetes have an increased numbers of glycoprotein IIb/IIIa receptors, which constitute the final common pathway for platelet activation when they bind with fibrinogen.

A consistent benefit of IIb/IIIa receptor antagonists in reducing ischaemic complications of non ST-segment elevation ACS has been demonstrated in a multiple trials. In a recent meta-analysis of trials evaluating the use of IIb/IIIa inhibitors in individuals with and without diabetes presenting with ACS, patients with diabetes not only had a reduction in ischaemic complications but a lower mortality. There was no such survival benefit in the group without diabetes. The decrease in mortality was predominantly among those patients with diabetes who underwent percutaneous coronary intervention.

6.2.2 **Anti-ischaemic therapy**
Beta-blockers are the preferred anti-ischemic drugs in acute coronary syndromes. Although data supporting a mortality benefit in patients with diabetes derive from sub-group analyses of patents with ST-segment elevation myocardial infarction, published guidelines recommend commencing beta-blockers in all patients with ACS in the absence of contra-indications. Despite the potential risks of worsening glycaemic control, masking hypoglycaemia and dyslipidaemias beta-blockers are generally well tolerated by patients with diabetes and coronary heart disease.

In addition (or as an alternative) to beta-blockers, nitrates, calcium channel blockers and nicorandil provide effective relief from ischaemic symptoms, although have not been shown to result in survival benefits in acute coronary syndromes.

6.2.3 **Anti-thrombotic therapy**
Unfractionated heparin (UFH) reduces the risk of death and myocardial infarction in patients with non ST-segment elevation ACS. Low molecular weight heparins (LMWH) eliminate the need for haematological monitoring and offer the advantage of simpler administration via the subcutaneous route. The LMWH enoxaparin has shown

superiority over UFH in the reduction of ischaemic events in clinical trials although has not been studied exclusively in patients with diabetes. The Factor Xa inhibitor fondaparinux reduces ischaemic events to a similar extent as enoxaparin, but is associated with a lower risk of major bleeding and lower mortality.

6.2.4 **Revascularization**

Patients with ACS and diabetes are at high risk for subsequent complications. Several randomized trails have compared medical therapy with an early invasive strategy (comprising coronary angiography and in-patient revascularization when appropriate) in patients presenting with non ST-segment elevation ACS. Pooled data from these studies demonstrate clinical benefit from an early invasive strategy, particularly in patients with moderate or high risk features. The magnitude of benefit is similar in patients with and without diabetes. However, as patients with diabetes are at higher absolute risk of adverse events, an early invasive approach confers a greater benefit in this group. The relative merits of percutaneous coronary intervention and coronary artery bypass grafting are discussed in Chapter 7.

6.3 **ST-segment elevation acute coronary syndromes**

6.3.1 **Initial treatment**

In patients with ST-segment elevation myocardial infarction, the presence of diabetes is associated with a greater risk of complications and higher short- and long-term mortality. Patients with diabetes present later, are more likely to have atypical symptoms, and more likely to present with cardiogenic shock than patients without diabetes. Despite the higher risk of adverse outcomes, individuals with diabetes are less likely to receive treatment according to established guidelines, particularly pharmacological reperfusion or mechanical reperfusion with percutaneous coronary intervention.

Aspirin produces a rapid anti-thrombotic effect by inhibiting production of thromboxane A2. In unselected patients with ST-segment elevation myocardial infarction, aspirin alone reduces mortality and confers additional benefit when given in combination with fibrinolytic agents.

Two recent randomized controlled trials have demonstrated additional benefits of clopidogrel when added to aspirin in patients with ST-segment myocardial infarction receiving fibrinolysis. The addition of clopidogrel improved infarct-related vessel patency, reduced re-infarction and improved mortality.

Dual oral antiplatelet therapy, with aspirin and a thienopyridine, is mandatory when percutaneous coronary intervention is chosen as the preferred reperfusion strategy.

6.3.2 **Fibrinolysis**

The initial goal in the management of ST-segment elevation myocardial infarction is to achieve reperfusion of the infarction-related artery and limit infarction size. The Fibrinolytic Therapy Trialists Collaborative group reviewed early adverse outcomes and mortality in nine large randomized trials of fibrinolytic therapy in 58,600 patients with suspected ST-segment elevation myocardial infarction. Mortality was reduced from 11.5% in the control group to 9.6% in patients recieving fibrinolysis. Although absolute mortality was higher in the 4,529 patients with diabetes, fibrinolysis conferred a greater reduction in mortality in this group (17.3% versus 13.6%).

Despite the clear mortality benefits, registry data demonstrate that patients with diabetes are less likely to receive fibrinolytic therapy than patients without diabetes. Atypical or late presentation to medical care, or unfounded concerns over haemorrhagic complications of fibrinolysis in patients with diabetes may contribute to this discrepancy.

6.3.3 **Primary percutaneous coronary intervention**

Primary percutaneous coronary intervention (PCI) for ST-segment elevation myocardial infarction yields more favourable outcomes than fibrinolytic therapy, with pooled analysis from randomized trials demonstrating significant reductions in all-cause mortality, non fatal re-infarction and stroke. A recent analysis of individual patient data from 19 trials of primary PCI versus fibrinolysis compared outcomes in patients with and without diabetes. Absolute 30-day mortality was higher in patients with diabetes. However, primary PCI was associated with similar reductions in mortality compared with fibrinolysis in patients with diabetes (relative risk reduction 51%) and those without diabetes (relative risk reduction 41%).

Primary PCI is now recommended as the preferred reperfusion strategy for ST-segment elevation myocardial infarction provided it can be delivered promptly by centres with experience in the technique.

6.3.4 **Early post-infarction management**

Treatment with beta-blockers reduces mortality in unselected patients following myocardial infarction. Sub-group analyses from randomized controlled trials demonstrate that beta-blockers are particularly effective in reducing mortality and recurrent myocardial infarction in patients with diabetes. In the absence of contraindications, oral beta-blockers are recommended for all patients with diabetes following myocardial infarction. Angiotensin converting enzyme inhibitors started in unselected patients within 24 hours of an ST-segment myocardial infarction reduce mortality and the risk of developing heart failure. The benefits are similar in patients with and without diabetes. Greater benefits are apparent in those with symptoms of heart failure or evidence of left ventricular systolic dysfunction. The angiotensin receptor blocker valsartan has been associated with an equivalent survival advantage to the angiotensin converting enzyme inhibitor captopril in high risk post-infarction patients with diabetes. In patients with heart failure post-myocardial infarction, the addition of the aldosterone antagonsist eplerenone reduces all cause mortality, cardiac mortality and re-hospitalization. These beneficial effects are consistent in patients with diabetes. However, the potential to induce hyperkalaemia may limit the use of eplerenone in patients with diabetes and microalbuminura.

6.4 **Management after acute coronary syndromes**

6.4.1 **Glycaemic control**

Random blood glucose levels in unselected patients admitted with ACS are strongly correlated with adverse short- and long-term outcomes. In patents with diabetes and ACS, high blood glucose levels are highly predictive of in-hospital and subsequent mortality. Data from trials testing a strategy of intensive glycaemic control in the immediate post-infarction period are conflicting. In the Diabetes, Glucose And Myocardial Infarction (DIGAMI) study, patients presenting with ACS and acute hyperglycaemia on admission were randomized to insulin-glucose infusion followed by subcutaneous insulin treatment or to conventional care. Mean blood glucose concentrations were 9.5 mmol/L in the intensive insulin-treated group and 11.6 mmol/L in the conventional treatment group. Mortality was reduced by 25% after 3.4 years of follow up in the intensive treatment group.

In the DIGAMI-2 study, 1,253 patients with type 2 diabetes and ACS were randomized to one of three treatment strategies: insulin-glucose infusion followed by long-term insulin-based glucose control, insulin-glucose infusion followed by standard glucose control, and routine management of blood glucose according to local practice. The study confirmed that glycaemic control is highly predictive of 2-year mortality but did not reveal any significant difference in outcomes between the three strategies of glycaemic control. However, these results must be interpreted in the context that fasting glucose levels in the first group did not reach target and no difference in long-term glycaemic control, assessed by HbA1c, was achieved between the three groups.

The Hyperglycemia Intensive Insulin Infusion in Infarction (HI-5) study randomized 240 patients with acute myocardial infarction to insulin/dextrose infusion, with a target blood glucose <10 mmol/L, or to conventional therapy. Again, blood glucose concentrations in the intensively treated group were not significantly lower than in the conventional treatment group. Insulin infusion failed to reduce the primary endpoint of mortality, but was associated with a lower incidence of cardiac failure and re-infarction within three months.

Post-infarction glycaemic control is specifically addressed in two recent Scientific Statements published by the American Heart Association and by the American Association of Clinical Endocrinologists/American Diabetes Association. These statements acknowledge the methodological limitations of previous trials and recommend further research in this area. However, both recommended treating glycaemia in patients with acute myocardial infarction and blood glucose of 10 mmol/L or higher with insulin therapy.

6.4.2 **Secondary prevention after ACS**

The high risk of recurrent events and increased mortality in patients with diabetes following ACS mandates an intensive approach to secondary prevention.

Although evidence suggests that aspirin may induce less effective platelet inhibition in individuals with diabetes, meta-analysis of secondary prevention trials confirms a consistent protective effect in sub-groups with diabetes. The addition of clopidogrel for up to 12 months following ACS further reduces ischaemic complications and mortality.

Beta-blockers are effective in reducing re-infarction and sudden death in patients with diabetes after myocardial infarction. Concerns over deterioration in glycaemic control or blunted counter-regulatory responses to hypoglycaemia rarely translate into clinically relevant problems.

Optimal secondary prevention also comprises intensive control of blood pressure and lipid profile, inhibition of the renin-angiotensin-aldosterone system and appropriate lifestyle measures including weight loss and smoking cessation. The roles of statins, angiotensin converting enzyme inhibitors, and angiotensin receptor blockers in secondary prevention in patients with diabetes and cardiovascular disease are discussed elsewhere in this book.

Unfortunately, despite the convincing evidence that secondary preventive measures reduce mortality in patients with coronary heart disease, most therapies are underutilised in patients with diabetes.

6.4.3 **Cardiac rehabilitation**

Cardiac rehabilitation is an important component of comprehensive care for patients following myocardial infarction. Rehabilitation programmes typically comprise exercise training, education and behavioural interventions. Their aim is to limit the physical and psychological effects of cardiac disease, reduce the risk of recurrent events and enhance the psychological and vocational status of participants. Cardiac rehabilitation programmes have been demonstrated to reduce all-cause mortality and improve symptoms, exercise capacity, well-being, lipid profiles and smoking cessation. The beneficial effects are consistent in participants with and without diabetes. The inclusion of diabetes-focussed multi-factorial interventions in a cardiac rehabilitation programme has recently been shown to lead to greater improvements in cardiovascular risk factors and glycaemic control.

6.5 **Conclusions**

Current data indicate that diabetes is common in patients presenting with ACS, confers a higher risk of mortality and recurrent cardiovascular events and is associated with a lower likelihood of receiving evidence-based therapies. Although advances in pharmacological and mechanical therapies have improved survival in patients with diabetes and ACS, outcomes remain impaired compared with individuals without diabetes.

References

Antithrombotic Trialists' Collaboration (2002) Collaborative meta-analysis of randomised trials of antiplatelet therapy for prevention of death, myocardial infarction, and stroke in high risk patients. *British Medical Journal* **324**: 71–86.

Cheung NW, Wong VW, McLean M (2006) The Hyperglycemia: Intensive Insulin Infusion in Infarction (HI-5) study: a randomized controlled trial of insulin infusion therapy for myocardial infarction. *Diabetes Care* **29**: 765–70.

Deedwania P, Kosiborod M, Barrett E, *et al.* American Heart Association Diabetes Committee of the Council on Nutrition, Physical Activity, and Metabolism (2008) Hyperglycemia and acute coronary syndrome: a scientific statement from the American Heart Association Diabetes Committee of the Council on Nutrition, Physical Activity, and Metabolism. *Circulation* **117**: 1610–19.

Malmberg K, Rydén L, Efendic S, *et al.* (1995) Randomized trial of insulin-glucose infusion followed by subcutaneous insulin treatment in diabetic patients with acute myocardial infarction (DIGAMI study): effects on mortality at 1 year. *Journal of the American College of Cardiology* **26**: 57–65.

Malmberg K, Rydén L, Wedel H, *et al.* (2005) Intense metabolic control by means of insulin in patients with diabetes mellitus and acute myocardial infarction (DIGAMI 2): effects on mortality and morbidity. *European Heart Journal* **26**: 650–61.

Moghissi ES, Korytkowski MT, Dinardo M, *et al.* American Association of Clinical Endocrinologists; American Diabetes Association (2009) American Association of Clinical Endocrinologists and American Diabetes

Association consensus statement on inpatient glycemic control. *Diabetes Care* **32**: 1191–1231.

Rydén L, Standl E, Bartnik M, *et al.* (2007) Guidelines on diabetes, pre-diabetes, and cardiovascular diseases: executive summary. The Task Force on Diabetes and Cardiovascular Diseases of the European Society of Cardiology (ESC) and of the European Association for the Study of Diabetes (EASD). *European Heart Journal* **28**: 88–136.

Timmer JR, Ottervanger JP, de Boer MJ, *et al.* Primary Coronary Angioplasty vs Thrombolysis-2 Trialists Collaborators Group (2007) Primary percutane-ous coronary intervention compared with fibrinolysis for myocardial infarc-tion in diabetes mellitus: results from the Primary Coronary Angioplasty vs Thrombolysis-2 trial. *Archives of Internal Medicine* **167**: 1353–9.

Yusuf S, Zhao F, Mehta SR, Chrolavicius S, Tognoni G, Fox KK; Clopidogrel in Unstable Angina to Prevent Recurrent Events Trial Investigators (2001) Effects of clopidogrel in addition to aspirin in patients with acute coronary syndromes without ST-segment elevation. *New England Journal of Medicine* **345**: 494–502.

Chapter 7

Coronary revascularization in the patient with diabetes

Owen Bebb and Stephen Wheatcroft

> **Key points**
> - Patients with diabetes represent a substantial proportion of patients undergoing coronary artery bypass graft (CABG) surgery and percutaneous coronary intervention (PCI)
> - The diffuse and rapidly progressive nature of coronary disease in individuals with diabetes pose significant challenges for revascularization
> - Despite recent technological advances in surgical and percutaneous techniques, clinical outcomes remain poorer for patients with diabetes compared to those without
> - Selection of revascularization strategy should be based on consideration of the severity and extent of coronary artery disease and the potential for complete revascularization
> - CABG offers advantages over PCI in individuals with diabetes and multi-vessel disease, with reduced requirement for repeat revascularization but no difference in survival.

7.1 Introduction

Individuals with diabetes have a greater prevalence of coronary atherosclerosis, with more diffuse disease, greater left-main stem and multi-vessel involvement and accelerated disease progression compared to those without diabetes. Patients with diabetes represent a significant proportion of those requiring coronary revascularization and present specific challenges for both coronary artery bypass graft

(CABG) surgery and percutaneous coronary intervention (PCI). Despite substantial improvements in both surgical and percutaneous techniques over the past decade, the outcomes of revascularization in patients with diabetes remain sub-optimal compared with individuals without diabetes.

7.2 Medical therapy or revascularization?

7.2.1 Background

The choice between medical therapy or revascularization in an individual patient is informed by many factors including clinical presentation, the severity and complexity of coronary disease, the presence of co-morbidities and physician/patient preference. In acute coronary syndromes, a strategy of invasive investigation proceeding to revascularization leads to improved outcomes, at least in higher risk individuals with elevated biomarkers of myocardial necrosis. For many patients with stable coronary disease, however, optimal medical therapy may be an appropriate initial strategy if symptoms are satisfactorily controlled. Historical trials suggested that revascularization with CABG offers a survival advantage over conservative management in patients with certain anatomical patterns of disease, including left-main coronary disease, or multi-vessel disease involving the proximal portion of the left anterior descending coronary artery when left ventricular function is impaired. More recently, randomized controlled trials have compared contemporary intensive medical management with revascularization with CABG or PCI in patients with diabetes and coronary artery disease.

7.2.2 Randomized trials of optimal medical therapy versus revascularization

In the COURAGE study, 2287 patients with coronary artery disease and evidence of ischaemia were randomized to optimal medical therapy or revascularization with PCI in addition to optimal medical therapy. Patients with left-main coronary disease, severe symptoms or markedly positive stress tests were excluded. Over a median follow-up of 4.6 years, PCI did not reduce the risk of death and non-fatal myocardial infarction. This negative result was consistent in patients with and without diabetes. A sub study of participants in the COURAGE trial who had undergone myocardial perfusion imaging, however, indicated a benefit from PCI in those patients with large areas of ischaemia.

The landmark BARI-2D study randomized 2,368 patients with diabetes and coronary artery disease to either prompt revascularisztion (CABG or PCI) with intensive medical therapy or intensive medical therapy alone. The decision about the type of revascularization was made on clinical grounds before randomization and was not part of the randomization process. In accordance with the factorial design of the BARI-2D study, participants were also randomized to receive insulin sensitizing or insulin providing strategy of glycaemic control. At five years, there were no differences in the primary outcome measures of death or freedom from major cardiovascular events between patients assigned to revascularization compared with those allocated intensive medical therapy alone. Survival was also similar in patients assigned to insulin-sensitization versus insulin provision therapy. Although there was no proven benefit from prompt revascularization in the trial as a whole, in patients allocated to the CABG stratum of the study, revascularization was associated with fewer major cardiovascular events than intensive medical therapy, driven by a significant reduction in risk of non-fatal myocardial infarction. It is unclear whether the apparent benefit from revascularization in this group is attributable to the more severe coronary disease in these patients or the type of revascularization.

Collectively, these trials suggest that an initial strategy of intensive medical therapy is reasonable for many patients with diabetes and coronary artery disease, but that revascularization may be appropriate in patients with large burden of ischaemia and/or more severe disease. It is also clear that revascularization may be required for limiting symptoms in medically treated patients, as there was substantial cross-over from the conservative to interventional arms of both the COURAGE and BARI-2D studies during follow-up.

7.3 Coronary artery bypass graft surgery

7.3.1 CABG in patients with diabetes

Individuals with diabetes represent up to a quarter of those undergoing CABG surgery. These individuals are often more unwell, older and have a higher prevalence of hypertension and heart failure than comparable patents without diabetes undergoing CABG. The surgical approach, which usually affords complete revascularization, is particularly appropriate in those with diabetes and multi-vessel involvement and/or left-main stem disease.

7.3.2 Diabetes and outcomes

Diabetes has been shown in some, but not all, studies to be an independent risk factor for early and late mortality following CABG. A number of diabetes-related factors have been linked to adverse outcomes, including:
- more severe coronary artery disease
- greater likelihood of left ventricular dysfunction

- increased neointimal hyperplasia resulting in graft occlusion
- increased risk of perioperative complications.

7.3.3 **Diabetes and peri-operative complications**

Table 7.1 summarizes common post-operative complications which are more frequent in patients with diabetes. Diabetes increases the risk of superficial sternal wound infections and mediastinitis, and infections of saphenous vein or radial artery harvest sites. Saphenous vein harvest site infections may be reduced in patients with diabetes by refinements in surgical technique, including endoscopic vein harvesting. Diabetes has also been shown to be an independent risk factor for renal failure and neurological complications including stroke. The relative risk of renal failure is five-fold higher in individuals with diabetes compared to patients without undergoing cardiac surgery. Low cardiac output syndrome is also more frequent in the presence of diabetes, suggesting that diabetes adversely affects myocardial function peri-operatively. Patients with diabetes undergoing CABG tend to stay longer on the intensive care unit post-operatively and have prolonged hospital stays, with a greater chance of re-admission, compared to patients without diabetes.

7.3.4 **Off-pump surgery**

In conventional CABG surgery, cardiopulmonary bypass is used to maintain perfusion whilst the heart is arrested for anastomosis of the bypass grafts. Recently, 'off-pump' or 'beating heart' surgery, in which anastomoses are fashioned without cardiopulmonary bypass, has become widely available. Off-pump CABG has been shown to reduce the likelihood of postoperative complications, including atrial fibrillation, renal failure, and respiratory failure, in patients with diabetes. Whether this translates in to a survival advantage for patients with diabetes undergoing off-pump CABG, however, is not yet clear.

Table 7.1 Complications associated with diabetes in patients undergoing cardiac surgery	
Infections	Sternal wound infections
	Mediastinitis
	Saphenous vein harvest site infection
Renal complications	Renal failure
	Requirement for dialysis
Neurological complications	Stroke
Haemodynamic complications	Low cardiac output syndrome

7.3.5 **Arterial revascularization**

The conduits typically employed for CABG include the long saphenous veins, internal mammary artery and radial artery. Saphenous vein conduits are prone to neointima formation, particularly in individuals with diabetes, pre-empting recurrent symptoms or graft occlusion. Arterial conduits, typically comprising internal mammary or radial arteries, are much less prone to restenosis and occlusion. In patients with diabetes undergoing CABG, the use of arterial grafts has been suggested to improve clinical outcomes including survival. The use of the left internal mammary artery for CABG has become standard practice, especially in patients with diabetes. The use of bilateral internal mammary arteries as conduits for grafting has been shown to be safe with a possible survival advantage in recent studies of patients with diabetes, but is avoided by some surgeons due to concerns over an increased risk of sternal wound infections.

7.3.6 **Post-operative care**

Intensive management of blood glucose levels with continuous insulin infusion has been shown to reduce morbidity and mortality in critically ill patients. A recent study of patients in the intensive care setting, the majority of whom had undergone cardiac surgery, showed a significant improvement in mortality with continuous insulin infusion. Other studies, showing reduced rates of sternal wound infection, support a policy of intensive glycaemic control in the post-operative period for patients with diabetes undergoing CABG.

7.4 **Percutaneous coronary intervention**

7.4.1 **Percutaneous coronary intervention in diabetic patients**

Patients with diabetes represent a substantial proportion of those undergoing percutaneous coronary intervention. Over the last two decades, the average age, lesion complexity and proportion presenting with unstable coronary disease have all increased in this group. Diabetes increases the risk of procedural complications, symptom recurrence, requirements for repeat revascularization and mortality in those undergoing PCI. Table 7.2 summarises factors contributing to these impaired outcomes.

7.4.2 **Balloon angioplasty**

Percutaneous Transluminal Coronary Angioplasty (PTCA) results in similar procedural success and early symptom relief in individuals with and without diabetes. However, diabetes substantially increases angiographic rates of restenosis and the requirement for

Table 7.2 **factors contributing to adverse outcomes following PCI in patients with diabetes**
Diffuse coronary artery disease
Increased prevalence of multi-vessel disease
Increased lesion calcification
Pro-thrombotic tendency
Resistance to anti-platelet drugs
Increased neointima formation
Increased risk of contrast-induced nephropathy

repeat revascularization for recurrent symptoms. A number of factors have been implicated in the unfavorable influence of diabetes on restenosis, including:

- exaggerated smooth muscle cell proliferation and hyperplasia
- advanced glycation end products
- inflammation
- growth factor production in response to hyperglycaemia
- endothelial dysfunction
- accelerated fibrosis and altered matrix components
- enhanced thrombogenicity
- increased elastic recoil.

These factors are compounded by the presence of longer, more complex stenoses and greater prevalence of multi-vessel disease in individuals with diabetes. Restenosis culminating in occlusion of the treated vessel is a strong independent predictor of long-term mortality in patients with diabetes.

7.4.3 **Coronary stents**

Over the last decade, implantation of coronary stents has become standard practice in the vast majority of PCI procedures. Stents facilitate greater acute luminal gain, provide a mechanical scaffold to prevent elastic recoil and reduce the effects of smooth muscle cell hyperplasia on luminal diameter. Multiple studies have shown that coronary stent deployment reduces restenosis compared to PTCA in individuals with and without diabetes. However, diabetes remains an important independent risk factor for restenosis in patients receiving coronary stents.

7.4.4 **Drug-eluting stents**

Drug eluting stents reduce restenosis by combining the mechanical scaffolding properties of a stent with drugs which inhibit vascular smooth cell proliferation and migration. Drugs such as paclitaxel or sirolimus (and related compounds) are typically bound to the stent struts with a polymer to facilitate controlled elution of the drug in a predictable manner after deployment. Initial clinical trials showed that drug eluting stents virtually abolished restenosis in highly selected coronary lesions. Contemporary trial and registry data from patients with a wide range of lesion types suggest that drug-eluting stents reduce the risk of restenosis by up to 70%. Although the absolute risk of restenosis remains higher in patients with diabetes, the relative reduction conferred by drug-eluting stents is preserved in the presence of diabetes.

The favorable effect of drug-eluting stents on restenosis risk has facilitated the rapid expansion of PCI to encompass treatment of increasingly more diffuse and complex types of coronary disease, including multi-vessel disease.

7.4.5 **Antiplatelet therapy**

The pro-thrombotic tendency associated with diabetes, which is an independently risk factor for stent thrombosis, mandates appropriate anti-platelet therapy following PCI. The use of combined oral antiplatelet drugs, typically comprising aspirin and a thienopyridine (ticlopidine, clopidogrel, or prasugrel) has become standard therapy to prevent immediate and late thrombotic complications of PCI. Recent trials have shown that adequate loading of these drugs prior to the interventional procedure reduces complications. Aspirin and a thienopyridine are usually continued for between one and twelve months following PCI, depending on the mode of presentation (stable or unstable) and type of stent (bare-metal or drug-eluting). In a recent sub-study of the Clopidogrel in Unstable angina to Reduce Recurrent Events (CURE) trial of patients with acute coronary syndromes undergoing PCI (PCI-CURE), dual antiplatelet therapy with aspirin and clopidogrel significantly reduced the risk of cardiovascular death or recurrent MI at one year in the subgroup with diabetes, compared with aspirin alone. The TRITON-TIMI 38 study further demonstrated that prasugrel offers additional protection from ischaemic cardiovascular events compared to clopidogrel in patients with diabetes undergoing PCI.

Intravenous glycoprotein IIb/IIIa inhibitors (abciximab, eptifibatide, and tirofiban) have been shown in multiple trials to reduce peri-procedural complications in high-risk patients undergoing PCI. Meta-analyses of trials reporting outcomes in sub-groups with diabetes demonstrate that abciximab reduced mortality by 45% at one year following PCI in patients with diabetes. The effect was most pronounced in insulin treated individuals and those receiving multiple stents. However, a more recent trial suggests that adequate pre-treatment with clopidogrel (600 mg at least 2 hours prior to the procedure) may negate the benefit of abciximab administration in stable patients with diabetes undergoing elective PCI. Intensive anti-platelet therapy, including intravenous glycoprotein IIb/IIIa inhibition, remains the standard of care in patients undergoing PCI for acute coronary syndromes. Although data specific to diabetes are lacking, the direct thrombin inhibitor bivalirudin, which inhibits platelets by reducing thrombin-mediated platelet activation, is emerging as an alternative to the combination of heparin and glycoprotein IIb/IIIa inhibitors during PCI.

7.4.6 **Peri-procedural care**

Contrast-induced nephropathy is not uncommon in patients undergoing PCI and portends a significant mortality and morbidity. Diabetes is an important risk factor for contrast-induced nephropa-thy, along with pre-existing renal disease, low cardiac output states and the volume of contrast used. Adequate pre-hydration and the use of iso-osmolar or non-ionic contrast agents may reduce the risk of contrast-induced nephropathy in individuals with diabetes and impaired renal function undergoing PCI. Data relating to the use of N-acetylcysteine for renal protection are conflicting. The only study carried out exclusively in patients with diabetes did not show a significant benefit.

Management of hyperglycaemia in patients with acute coronary syn-dromes is discussed in Chapter 6. In the setting of elective PCI, opti-mal glycaemic control is associated with lower rates of target vessel revascularization in patients with type 2 diabetes. Metformin, how-ever, is conventionally withheld from patients undergoing PCI peri-procedurally, due to the rare possibility of metformin accumulation in patients who develop renal failure precipitating lactic acidosis.

7.5 **Percutaneous coronary intervention versus coronary artery bypass grafting**

7.5.1 **Choice of revascularization strategy**

Despite recent advances in both surgical and percutaneous tech-niques, patients with diabetes present specific challenges to both interventional cardiologists and cardiac surgeons undertaking coro-nary revascularization. A number of factors may influence the deci-sion of whether surgical or percutaneous revascularization is chosen for an individual patient. These include the number of diseased ves-sels (including left main coronary artery involvement), left ventricu-lar function and the presence or absence of co-morbidities which may increase peri-procedural risk. As discussed below, several ran-domized controlled trials have compared CABG with PCI in patients with diabetes and multi-vessel disease.

7.5.2 **CABG versus balloon angioplasty**

The Bypass Angioplasty Revascularization (BARI) trial randomized 1829 patients with multi-vessel disease to either balloon angioplasty or CABG. There was no difference in survival according to revascularization strategy for the trial as a whole. However, in those with diabetes (353 patients), seven-year survival was substantially higher in the CABG group than in the angioplasty group (76.4% versus 55.7%). These findings led a number of organizations to recommend that CABG should be considered the revascularization strategy of choice for patients with diabetes. Subsequent analyses of the BARI trial suggested that survival advantage conferred by CABG was limited to patients who underwent arterial revascularization using an internal mammary artery graft, and that the mortality benefit was most apparent in those experiencing a myocardial infarction during follow-up. However, in a registry of patients with diabetes who were screened for the BARI study but not entered into the randomized trial, there was no difference in survival between those receiving CABG or angioplasty. Similarly, other randomized trials in the balloon angioplasty era did not corroborate the mortality advantage conferred by CABG in the BARI trial (Table 7.3).

7.5.3 **CABG versus coronary stent deployment**

Several randomized trials comparing CABG with coronary stent deployment for multi-vessel disease provide outcome data for subgroups with diabetes (Table 7.4). In the Arterial Revascularization Therapies Study (ARTS), 208 patients with diabetes and multi-vessel disease underwent CABG or PCI with stent deployment. Mortality was not significantly different between the surgical or percutaneous approaches but freedom from clinical events was lower in the PCI group (63.4% versus 84%), almost entirely due to an increased requirement for target vessel revascularization in those undergoing PCI. The 150 patients with diabetes in the Stents or Surgery (SOS) trial had no difference in mortality according to treatment strategy. The Angina With Extremely Serious Operative Mortality Evaluation

Table 7.3 Selected trials of angioplasty versus **CABG** for multi-vessel disease in patients with diabetes

Trial	Patients (n)	Follow-up (years)	Mortality (%)		P-value
			CABG	PCI	
BARI	353	7	23.6	44.3	<0.001
CABRI	124	4	12.5	22.6	ns
EAST	59	8	24.5	39.9	ns
BARI-registry	339	5	14.9	14.4	ns

Table 7.4 Selected trials of stents versus CABG for multi-vessel disease in patients with diabetes

Trial	Patients (n)	Follow-up (years)	Mortality (%)		P-value
			CABG	PCI	
ARTS	208	3	4.2	7.1	0.39
SoS	150	1	0.8	2.5	ns
AWESOME	144	5	34	26	0.27
SYNTAX	452	1	6.4	8.4	0.43
CARDIA	510	1	3.2	3.2	0.97

(AWESOME) randomized 454 high risk patients requiring revascularization to CABG or PCI. 144 patents had diabetes and the majority (although not all) of individuals randomized to PCI underwent stent deployment. Mortality was similar in patients with diabetes treated by CABG or PCI. These studies compared CABG with the deployment of bare-metal coronary stents, which are prone to restenosis in patients with diabetes.

More recent studies have investigated whether PCI with drug-eluting stents offers similar outcomes to those achieved with surgery. The SYNTAX trial randomized 1800 patients with left main and/or three-vessel coronary disease to CABG or PCI with paclitaxel-eluting stents. In the 452 patients with medically-treated diabetes, the study revealed a higher incidence of major adverse cardiac and

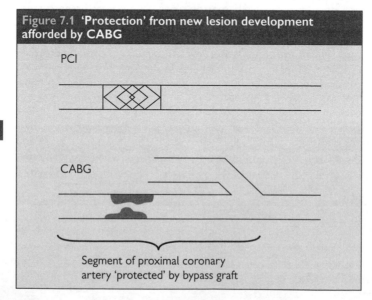

Figure 7.1 'Protection' from new lesion development afforded by CABG

PCI

CABG

Segment of proximal coronary
artery 'protected' by bypass graft

cerebrovascular events, including death, stroke, myocardial infarction and repeat revascularization, associated with PCI compared with CABG. Consistent with the SYNTAX trial as a whole, the difference was driven by a higher rate of repeat revascularization in the PCI group. The incidence of death, stroke and myocardial infarction in patients with diabetes was similar whether they received CABG or PCI. The CARDIA study was the first diabetes-specific coronary revascularization trial in which 510 patients with multivessel or complex single-vessel coronary artery disease were allocated to CABG or PCI with either bare-metal or sirolimus-eluting stents. The results failed to demonstrate that PCI is non-inferior to CABG, and again revealed significantly higher rates of repeat revascularization in patients treated with PCI.

The balance of evidence, therefore, suggests that PCI with stent deployment affords comparable survival to CABG in patients with diabetes and multi-vessel disease, but that the requirement for repeat revascularization is higher with PCI compared with CABG.

The reduced requirements for repeat revascularization following CABG may be due to the fact that bypass grafts can maintain distal coronary perfusion even if new stenoses develop in the proximal vessel. Coronary stents, being a focal treatment, cannot 'protect' against de novo lesion development in untreated coronary segments. This difference may be exaggerated by the progressive nature of atherosclerosis in individuals with diabetes. See also Figure 7.1.

7.6 **Conclusions**

The diffuse and rapidly progressive nature of coronary artery disease in individuals with diabetes presents significant challenges for revascularization. Despite ongoing technological refinements in surgical and percutaneous techniques, outcomes remain suboptimal compared to those without diabetes. An initial strategy of intensive medical therapy is appropriate for many patients with diabetes and coronary artery disease. When revascularization is indicated, selection of the most appropriate modality should be based on consideration of the severity and extent of coronary artery disease and the potential for complete revascularization. Current evidence suggests that contemporary PCI and CABG offer comparable survival in patients with diabetes. However, CABG offers advantages compared to PCI in multi-vessel disease due to the greater freedom from angina and lower requirement for repeat revascularization.

References

Abizaid A, Costa MA, Centemero M, et al., the ARTS investigators (2001) Clinical and economic impact of diabetes mellitus on percutaneous and surgical treatment of multivessel coronary disease patients. Insights from the Arterial Revascularization Therapy Study. *Circulation* **104**: 533–8.

Banning AP, Westaby S, Morice MC, *et al.* (2010) Diabetic and nondiabetic patients with left main and/or 3-vessel coronary artery disease: comparison of outcomes with cardiac surgery and paclitaxel-eluting stents. *Journal of the American College of Cardiology* **55**: 1067–75.

BARI 2D Study Group, Frye RL, August P, Brooks MM, *et al.* (2009) A randomized trial of therapies for type 2 diabetes and coronary artery disease. *New England Journal of Medicine* **360**: 2503–15.

The BARI Investigators (2000) Seven year outcome in the bypass angioplasty revascularisation investigation (BARI) by treatment and diabetic status. *Journal of the American College of Cardiology* **35**: 1122–29.

Berry C, Tardif JC, Bourassa MG (2007) Coronary heart disease in patients with diabetes: part II: recent advances in coronary revascularization. *Journal of the American College of Cardiology* **49**: 643–56.

Boden WE, O'Rourke RA, Teo KK, *et al.*, COURAGE Trial Research Group (2007) Optimal medical therapy with or without PCI for stable coronary disease. *New England Journal of Medicine* **356**: 1503–16.

Bravata DM, Gienger AL, McDonald KM, *et al.* (2007) Systematic review: the comparative effectiveness of percutaneous coronary interventions and coronary artery bypass graft surgery. *Annals of Internal Medicine* **147**: 703–16.

Chaitman BR, Hardison RM, Adler D, *et al.*, Bypass Angioplasty Revascularization Investigation 2 Diabetes (BARI 2D) Study Group (2009) The Bypass Angioplasty Revascularization Investigation 2 Diabetes randomized trial of different treatment strategies in type 2 diabetes mellitus with stable ischemic heart disease: impact of treatment strategy on cardiac mortality and myocardial infarction. *Circulation* **120**(25): 2529–40. Erratum in: (2010) *Circulation* **121**: e254.

Kapur A, Hall RJ, Malik IS, *et al.* (2010) Randomized comparison of percutaneous coronary intervention with coronary artery bypass grafting in diabetic patients. 1-year results of the CARDia (Coronary Artery Revascularization in Diabetes) trial. *Journal of the American College of Cardiology* **55**: 432–40.

Shaw LJ, Berman DS, Maron DJ, *et al.*, COURAGE Investigators (2008) Optimal medical therapy with or without percutaneous coronary intervention to reduce ischemic burden: results from the Clinical Outcomes Utilizing Revascularization and Aggressive Drug Evaluation (COURAGE) trial nuclear substudy. *Circulation* **117**: 1283–91.

Stone KE, Chiquette E, Chilton RJ (2007) Diabetic endovascular disease: role of coronary artery revascularization. *American Journal of Cardiology* **99**: 105B–112B.

Chapter 8

Chronic heart failure in diabetes

Miles Fisher

Key points

- Heart failure is common in people with diabetes, and diabetes is common in people with heart failure
- Coronary heart disease and previous myocardial infarction contribute to heart failure in people with diabetes, and a diabetic cardiomyopathy is also important
- Diastolic dysfunction is common in diabetes and may be the first sign of heart failure
- Most of the therapies that are proven to reduce mortality in patients with heart failure are of proven benefit in diabetes. There are few particular considerations on the use of beta-blockers
- The development of heart failure will require consideration of the most appropriate anti-diabetic drugs. Glitazones are contraindicated in heart failure but metformin can be used except during episodes of acute heart failure.

8.1 Epidemiology of heart failure in diabetes

Heart failure is the inability of the heart to pump sufficient oxygenated blood to the metabolizing tissues despite an adequate filling pressure. Chronic heart failure (CHF) can be caused by several types of cardiac dysfunction and is most commonly attributable to left ventricular systolic dysfunction (LVSD). CHF can also occur in the presence of preserved systolic function, and may be attributed to diastolic dysfunction.

Box 8.1 Risk factors for the development of congestive heart failure in diabetes

- Age
- Duration of diabetes
- Raised HbA1c
- Insulin use
- Increased body mass index
- Hypertension
- Previous coronary heart disease
- Retinopathy
- Urinary albumin excretion/proteinuria
- Nephropathy/end-stage renal disease

Diabetes is an independent risk factor for the development of CHF, and in the Framingham study diabetes increased the risk of CHF by twofold for men and fivefold for women. There are many risk factors for the development of CHF in people with diabetes (Box 8.1), and the most important of these are hypertension and previous coronary heart disease. Around 12% of patients with diabetes in population studies have CHF, rising to 22% in patients aged over 65 years. In people with LVSD the prevalence of diabetes ranges from 6–25%, increasing to 12–30% in patients with symptomatic CHF.

CHF carries a very poor prognosis, and diabetes is an independent predictor of mortality. Diabetic patients with CHF have a higher mortality rate and rate of hospitalisation compared to non-diabetic patients with CHF.

8.2 Mechanisms of heart failure in diabetes

Coronary heart disease and previous myocardial infarction both contribute to chronic heart failure in diabetes. Haemochromatosis can cause both diabetes and CHF. There is also a 'diabetic cardio-myopathy' that can impair systolic emptying or diastolic filling of the left ventricle, and contributes along with coronary heart disease to the high prevalence of CHF that is seen in people with diabetes. Several factors contribute to this cardiomyopathy, including bio-chemical and pathological changes in the myocardium and blood vessels (Box 8.2).

The neurendocrine responses to heart failure include activation of the renin-angiotensin-aldosterone system, activation of the sympathetic nervous system, raised serum cortisol and growth hormone. There are also increases in cytokines such as TNF-alpha, IL-1 and IL-6. As exercise tolerance worsens, physical activity declines and insulin

> **Box 8.2 Factors contributing to chronic heart failure in diabetes**
>
> **Higher prevalence of conditions associated with heart failure**
>
> - Coronary heart disease
> - Hypertension
> - Obesity
>
> **Other pathologies**
>
> - Diabetic cardiomyopathy
>   - myocardial fibrosis
>   - left ventricular hypertrophy
>   - endothelial changes and dysfunction
> - Diabetic cardiovascular autonomic neuropathy
>
> **Metabolic abnormalities**
>
> - Hyperglycaemia
> - Increased free fatty acids
> - Insulin resistance

resistance increases, leading to new onset diabetes. Interestingly, new onset diabetes is more likely to occur during treatment of CHF with metoprolol than during treatment with carvedilol.

8.3 Investigation of heart failure in diabetic patients

The diagnosis of chronic heart failure comprises a constellation of symptoms, signs, and the results of investigations:

- Symptoms include breathlessness, fatigue and ankle swelling. Symptoms are used to classify heart failure in the New York Heart Association (NYHA) classification
- Diabetic patients should be examined for the presence of clinical signs of CHF and for the complications of diabetes
- Biochemical testing includes iron studies, HbA1c, renal function, and urine examination for microalbuminuria or proteinuria. Measurement of BNP, where available, is useful in people with diabetes
- An ECG should be performed looking for previous silent myocardial infarction
- To confirm the diagnosis of CHF cardiac dysfunction must be demonstrated. Echocardiography will give an estimate of left

ventricular ejection fraction as a measure of systolic function, diastolic dysfunction, can identify wall motion abnormalities of coronary heart disease or previous myocardial infarction, and can exclude valvular and other forms of heart disease.

8.4 **Treatment of heart failure in diabetic patients**

The approach to the treatment of chronic heart failure is similar in diabetic and non-diabetic patients, and should include the use of diuretics, angiotensin-converting enzyme inhibitors (ACE inhibitors) or angiotensin-II receptor antagonists (ARAs), and beta-blockers. CHF causes neurohormonal activation, and neurohormonal block-ade with ACE inhibitors or ARBs and beta-blockers are the foun-dation of pharmacological therapy for CHF. Beta-blocker therapy should not be withheld in diabetic patients because of fears of hypoglycaemia.

8.4.1 **Diuretics**

Loop diuretics reduce fluid overload in patients with CHF and improve symptoms but do not appear to improve prognosis. Older studies suggested that bumetanide had less adverse effect on glu-cose tolerance than furosemide, but the evidence for this in people with diabetes is minimal and either drug can be used.

In one study the aldosterone antagonist spironolactone was added to diuretics, digoxin and ACE inhibitors in patients with LVSD and severe symptomatic CHF. Mortality was reduced by 30% overall. One quarter of the patients had diabetes and the reduc-tion in patients with diabetes was very similar. If this combination of spironolactone and ACE inhibitors is used in clinical practice there needs to be close monitoring of serum potassium and renal function in diabetic patients.

Eplerenone is a newer aldosterone antagonist that was studied following myocardial infarction in patients with LVSD and symptom-atic heart failure, or diabetic patients with LVSD (one third of the study subjects). Total mortality was reduced with eplerenone, and the benefit in patients with diabetes was similar. A study of epler-enone in patients with mild to moderate heart failure was stopped early because of a significant reduction in deaths and hospitalizations for heart failure. One third of the subjects had diabetes and the ben-efits were similar in diabetic and non-diabetic patients.

8.4.2 **ACE inhibitors and ARAs**

ACE inhibitors improve the prognosis in left ventricular systolic dys-function and CHF, and have been studied in several large multi-centre trials which have contained large numbers of subjects with diabetes.

Some have published separate subgroup analysis for diabetes and have shown very similar reductions in mortality in diabetic patients with CHF. In a large meta-analysis of over ten thousand subjects in four CHF trials and three trials of post-MI ventricular dysfunction a quarter of the patients had diabetes. ACE inhibitors reduced mortality by 14% in diabetic patients and 15% in non-diabetic subjects. Reductions were also seen in heart failure hospitalizations, and re-infarctions in patients with previous myocardial infarction with ACE inhibitors.

ARAs are an alternative to ACE inhibitors in patients that cannot tolerate ACE inhibitors because of cough, including patients with diabetes. Studies comparing ARAs and ACE inhibitors have shown conflicting results, as have studies combining ACE inhibitors and ARAs, and this combination is not routinely recommended for CHF treatment. There have been no separate published diabetes subgroup analyses for trials with ARAs, but within each study there has been no heterogeneity of effect in people with diabetes.

8.4.3 **Beta-blockers**

Beta-blockers have been studied in several large studies and reduce mortality in CHF. The studies included many diabetic patients, ranging from 12% to 29% of subjects, and subgroup analysis has shown similar benefits in people with diabetes and CHF. Despite this enormous evidence base, data from registers consistently shows that people with diabetes and CHF are less likely to be receiving beta-blocker therapy than non-diabetic patients. This has been attributed to misguided concerns about hypoglycaemia

The physiological response to hypoglycaemia includes activation of the autonomic nervous system. Epinephrine and norepinephrine stimulate glycogen breakdown to restore blood glucose concentrations to normal. This mechanism may be antagonised by non-selective beta-blockade, prolonging the recovery from hypoglycaemia. Non-selective beta-blockade may also slightly alter the autonomic symptomatic response to hypoglycaemia. For diabetic patients with CHF these are of only minor consequence as:

- Diabetic patients with CHF are often insulin resistant with poor glycaemic control, and the incidence of hypoglycaemia is low

- The cardioselective beta-blockers bisoprolol and metoprolol can be used for the treatment of CHF

- As described, the use of beta-blockers in diabetic patients with CHF has demonstrated beyond all doubt a reduction in total mortality and heart failure hositalization.

All patients with diabetes, LVSD and CHF should be considered for beta-blockers in addition to ACE inhibitors, and as for non-diabetic subjects they should be used with caution in patients with bradycardia, hypotension, or chronic obstructive pulmonary disease.

8.4.4 **Other drugs**

Several other drugs have been studied in people with CHF including digoxin, nitrates and hydralazine, but diabetic subgroup analysis is not available from these studies. In a recent study ivabradine reduced hospitalizations with heart failure and death from heart failure in patients with symptomatic heart failure and low ejection fractions. One third of the subjects had diabetes, and the benefits were similar in diabetic and non-diabetic patients.

8.4.5 **Device therapy in diabetic CHF**

Cardiac resynchronisation therapy pacing, also known as multi-site pacing or biventricular pacing, improves symptoms and prognosis in patients who have severe symptomatic CHF. Little diabetes data has been reported, but in two small studies diabetes subgroup analysis has shown similar improvements in morbidity and mortality in patients with and without diabetes.

There is also little specific data at present on the use of implantable cardiac defibrillators (ICDs) in diabetes. In one study no benefit was observed in a diabetes subgroup, and further research in diabetic patients is required.

8.4.6 **Surgery including cardiac transplantation**

Occasionally coronary interventions are used to improve the myocardial blood supply in patients with CHF. Cardiac transplantation is a possible treatment for patients who remain symptomatic despite optimal medical and device therapy, although the numbers of cardiac transplants performed has fallen since the widespread use of ACE inhibitors and beta-blockers in CHF. At first diabetes was a contraindication to transplantation, but excellent results can be obtained in selected diabetic patients. Active infection, e.g. diabetic foot ulceration is a contraindication because of the immunosupression that is required following cardiac transplantation. Large doses of steroids are used, worsening hyperglycaemia in diabetic patients, and leading to new-onset diabetes in many subjects that were previously non-diabetic.

8.5 **Treatment of diabetes in patients with heart failure**

The management of hyperglycaemia in diabetic patients is described in Chapter 2. Patients with CHF often have poor glycaemic control and require combinations of anti-diabetic drugs to try and improve control. There is no evidence that treatment of hyperglycaemia improves prognosis once CHF is present.

8.5.1 **Metformin**

Chronic heart failure was previously considered as a contraindication to metformin therapy, and it was thought that heart failure increased the risk of lactic acidosis with metformin. This has now been challenged on several grounds:

- The incidence of lactic acidosis with metformin is very low
- In case reports of lactic acidosis with metformin most have at least one other disease or illness that can result in lactic acidosis
- A Cochrane review of 176 trials showed similar rates of lactic acidosis between metformin and other oral antidiabetic drugs
- Large retrospective cohort studies examining the use of metformin in patients with CHF reported either no cases of lactic acidosis, or rates of lactic acidosis that were similar to those in patients not treated with metformin
- Large retrospective cohort studies of patients with diabetes and CHF have demonstrated that outcomes were *better* in patients on metformin compared to other antidiabetic therapies, with reductions in total mortality and reduced readmissions with heart failure (Figure 8.1).

Registry studies show that despite the contraindication metformin is frequently prescribed in patients with CHF. A pragmatic approach is to use metformin in stable heart failure (NYHA classes I and II), and to withdraw metformin during episodes of cardiac decompensation, when lactate production can be increased as a result of tissue hypoxia.

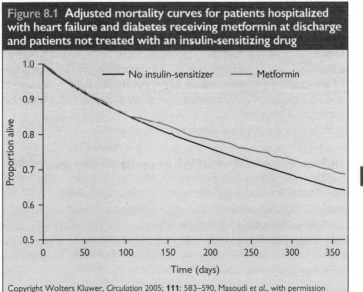

Figure 8.1 **Adjusted mortality curves for patients hospitalized with heart failure and diabetes receiving metformin at discharge and patients not treated with an insulin-sensitizing drug**

— No insulin-sensitizer — Metformin

Proportion alive

Time (days)

Copyright Wolters Kluwer, *Circulation* 2005; **111**: 583–590, Masoudi *et al.*, with permission

Box 8.3 Risk factors for the development of heart failure with glitazone treatment

- Previous chronic heart failure
- Previous myocardial infarction or stable coronary heart disease
- Hypertension
- Left ventricular hypertrophy
- Significant aortic or mitral valve disease
- Age over 70 years
- Duration of diabetes over 10 years
- Chronic renal failure
- Combination therapy with insulin

8.5.2 **Glitazones**

As described in Chapter 2 glitazones cause the retention of fluid through mechanisms in the distal tubules of the kidney. This may manifest itself as weight gain or ankle oedema. In a patient with early left ventricular systolic function, or diastolic dysfunction, this fluid retention can unmask heart failure, and glitazones are currently contra-indicated in patients with a history of chronic heart failure. There are several risk factors for the development of heart failure with glitazone therapy (Box 8.3).

This contraindication has also been challenged on the following grounds:

- Mechanistic studies have shown improvements in myocardial insulin-stimulated glucose uptake with glitazones, with no change in left ventricular ejection fraction on echocardiography
- In the PROactive study admissions with heart failure were increased but there was no increase in mortality or morbidity
- Meta-analysis of randomized clinical trails demonstrated increased heart failure events but no change in cardiovascular deaths (Figure 8.2), suggesting that heart failure in patients given glitazones might not carry the same risk that is seen in CHF caused by progressive ventricular dysfunction
- A large retrospective cohort study of patients with diabetes and CHF demonstrated a reduction in total mortality in patients pre-scribed glitazones, but increased readmissions with heart failure (Figure 8.3).

For the time being CHF remains a contraindication to glitazone therapy. If a patient develops fluid retention after starting pioglitazone they should be investigated for CHF as described in Section 8.3. If CHF is confirmed pioglitazone should be discontinued, but in the absence of left ventricular dysfunction pioglitazone can be continued.

Figure 8.2 Comparison of risk of congestive heart failure (A) and cardiovascular death (B) for rosiglitazone and pioglitazone

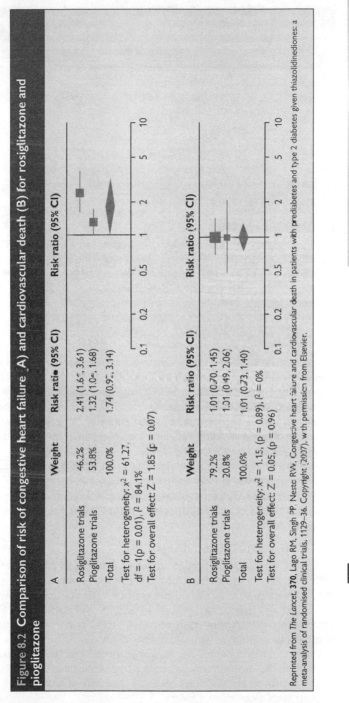

A	Weight	Risk ratio (95% CI)	Risk ratio (95% CI)
Rosiglitazone trials	46.2%	2.41 (1.61, 3.61)	
Pioglitazone trials	53.8%	1.32 (1.04, 1.68)	
Total	100.0%	1.74 (0.97, 3.14)	

Test for heterogeneity: $\chi^2 = 61.27$, df = 1(p = 0.01), $I^2 = 84.1\%$
Test for overall effect: Z = 1.85 (p = 0.07)

B	Weight	Risk ratio (95% CI)	Risk ratio (95% CI)
Rosiglitazone trials	79.2%	1.01 (0.70, 1.45)	
Pioglitazone trials	20.8%	1.01 (0.49, 2.06)	
Total	100.0%	1.01 (0.73, 1.40)	

Test for heterogeneity: $\chi^2 = 1.15$, (p = 0.89), $I^2 = 0\%$
Test for overall effect: Z = 0.05, (p = 0.96)

Reprinted from The Lancet, 370, Lago RM, Singh PP, Nesto RW, Congestive heart failure and cardiovascular death in patients with prediabetes and type 2 diabetes given thiazolidinediones: a meta-analysis of randomised clinical trials, 1129–36. Copyright 2007, with permission from Elsevier.

Figure 8.3 Adjusted mortality curves for patients hospitalized with heart failure and diabetes receiving a thiazolidinedione (TZD) at discharge and patients not treated with an insulin-sensitizing drug

Copyright Wolters Kluwer, *Circulation* 2005; **111**: 583–590, Masoudi *et al.*, with permission

8.5.3 **Insulin**

In some studies insulin use has been an independent predictor of mortality in diabetic patients with CHF. It is likely that insulin use is a marker either for patients with a long duration of diabetes and extensive cardiovascular disease, or that insulin is required when other treatments are ineffective in patients with severe CHF who have neurohormonal activation that worsens insulin resistance and hyperglycaemia.

Fluid retention is a rare side effect of insulin, occurring at the start of insulin therapy in poorly controlled patients. It is caused by the direct effect of insulin on sodium and water retention in the renal tubules, and may occasionally provoke symptomatic heart failure in patients with LVSD.

8.5.4 **Other antidiabetic drugs**

There are no contraindications to sulphonylureas in patients with CHF, but these may not control hyperglycaemia when used in isolation. There is little published experience with acarbose, or with the newer antidiabetic drugs such as DPP-4 inhibitors and GLP-1 receptor agonists. A pilot study of native GLP-1 given intravenously demonstrated improvements in ejection fraction in patients with left ventricular dysfunction following myocardial infarction. Another pilot study showed that continuous subcutaneous infusion of native GLP-1 improved ejection fraction and symptoms of heart failure in patients with chronic heart failure.

8.6 Conclusions

Chronic heart failure is common in patients with diabetes and can be treated in a similar way to heart failure in the non-diabetic patient. The best method of treating hyperglycaemia in heart failure patients, and the risk: benefit ratios of metformin and glitazones, require further research.

References

Bell DSH (2003) Diabetic cardiomyopathy. *Diabetes Care* **26**: 2949–51.

Lago RM, Singh PP, Nesto RW (2007) Congestive heart failure and cardiovascular death in patients with prediabetes and type 2 diabetes given thiazolidinediones: a meta-analysis of randomised clinical trials. *Lancet* **370**: 1129–36.

Macdonald MR, Petrie MC, McMurray JJ (2007) Diabetes, left ventricular systolic dysfunction and chronic heart failure. In: M Fisher and JJ McMurray, eds. *Diabetic cardiology*, pp. 93–134, John Wiley & Sons, Ltd, Chichester, UK.

Masoudi FA, Inzucchi SE, Wang Y, Havranek EP, Foody JM, Krumholz HM (2005) Thiazolidinediones, metformin, and outcomes in older patients with diabetes and heart failure: an observational study. *Circulation* **111**: 583–90.

Masoudi FA, Inzucchi SE (2007) Diabetes mellitus and heart failure: epidemiology, mechanisms, and pharmacotherapy. *American Journal of Cardiology* **99**(suppl): 113B–32B.

Tahrani AA, Varughese GI, Scarpello JH, Hanna FWF (2007) Metformin, heart failure, and lactic acidosis: is metformin absolutely contraindicated? *British Medical Journal* **335**: 508–12.

Chapter 9

Other vascular disease in diabetes

Miles Fisher

Key points

- Strokes are a common cause of morbidity in people with diabetes. Several secondary preventive therapies, including control of hypertension, statins, pioglitazone and the use of antiplatelet drugs are of benefit, but intensive management of hyperglycaemia in acute stroke carries no benefit
- Peripheral arterial disease is a common cause of morbidity in people with diabetes, and contributes to diabetic foot problems. Revascularization and some medical therapies may be helpful
- Erectile dysfunction is strongly associated with cardio-vascular disease in men with diabetes, and carries a poor prognosis
- Renovascular disease is increased in people with diabetes, and clinically has to be distinguished from other forms of diabetic kidney disease.

9.1 Introduction

Chapters 5–8 describe the consequences of coronary heart disease in diabetes, causing stable coronary heart disease, acute coronary syndromes, and chronic heart failure, which are common causes of death in people with diabetes. Other manifestations of atherosclerotic disease are common causes of morbidity in people with diabetes, including cerebrovascular disease, peripheral vascular disease, and erectile dysfunction.

Many studies of risk factor reduction have 'major cardiovascular disease', as one of the important endpoints, which comprises cardiovascular death, non-fatal myocardial infarction and non-fatal stroke.

Some studies will include cerebrovascular or peripheral vascular events as part of a composite end-point (Figure 9.1). As an example the primary endpoint in the PROactive study was a composite consisting of all cause mortality, non-fatal myocardial infarction, stroke, major leg amputation, acute coronary syndrome, cardiac intervention

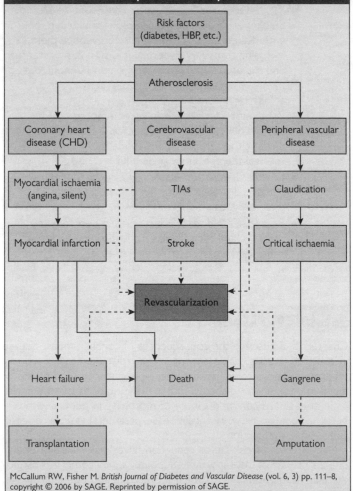

Figure 9.1 Natural history and outcomes of cardiovascular disease in different vascular beds. Some of the end points (full lines) are related to the progression of the disease, or so called "disease endpoints", and some are related to clinical decisions about admission or intervention (broken lines) or "procedure endpoints". Many composite outcomes will be a mixture of disease and procedure endpoints

McCallum RW, Fisher M. *British Journal of Diabetes and Vascular Disease* (vol. 6, 3) pp. 111–8, copyright © 2006 by SAGE. Reprinted by permission of SAGE.

including coronary artery bypass grafting or percutaneous coronary intervention, or leg revascularization.

It is well recognized that patients with atheroma in one vascular territory often have disease in other territories. In the Reduction of Atherothrombosis for Continued Health (REACH) registry of 67,888 patients with established arterial disease or high cardiovascular risk, of whom 44% had diabetes, one sixth of the patients with coronary artery disease, cerebrovascular disease (CVD) or peripheral arterial disease (PAD) had symptomatic involvement in two or three arterial beds, confirming the diffuse nature of atherothrombosis. Many also had asymptomatic disease elsewhere. On follow-up at one year the event rate increased according to the number of affected vascular beds, and was higher in diabetic than nondiabetic subjects.

9.2 Strokes and transient ischaemic attacks

Transient ischaemic attacks (TIAs) are classically transient neurological dysfunction lasting less than 24 hours and strokes are neurological dysfunction persisting for more than 24 hours. The risk of ischaemic stroke is increased three-fold in diabetes, and encompasses a spectrum of disease from large-vessel to small-vessel occlusive disease, which may be clinically symptomatic or asymptomatic and 'silent'. There dose not appear to be any increase in haemorrhagic stroke in diabetes.

9.2.1 Pathology

In patients with diabetes there is accelerated atherothrombotic change in the large extra-cranial carotid arteries. Diabetes also increases atheroma formation in large, medium and smaller arteries and arterioles of the cerebral circulation. In small intraparenchymal vessels there is an increase in 'microatheroma', basement membrane thickening, lipid deposition in the vessel wall and endothelial proliferation. These pathological changes cause vessel occlusion within the microcirculation, increasing the risk of lacunar infarction in the territory of single deep perforating arteries.

Lacunar infarction is more common in people with diabetes, and has a good prognosis for survival, but a high-risk of recurrence within the first year. Half of patients with a lacunar stroke will have persisting disability one year after the initial event.

9.2.2 Management of acute stroke in diabetes

Thrombolysis with alteplase given within four and a half hours of symptom onset of acute ischaemic stroke improves functional recovery. Hyperglycaemia may affect the response, and in one study admission hyperglycaemia was associated with a reduced chance of good clinical outcomes and a higher risk of intracranial haemorrhage following thrombolysis. In one observational series plasma glucose >11.2 mmol/l at the time of thrombolysis was associated with a five-fold increase in the risk of intracranial haemorrhage. Some guidelines have blood glucose <2.2 or >22 mmol/l as contraindications to thrombolysis in stroke.

9.2.3 Management of hyperglycaemia following stroke

Hyperglycaemia in patients with stroke carries a poor prognosis, both in diabetic patients and in patients with 'post stroke hyperglycaemia'. This may be because of lactate accumulation and a lower survival of cells in the potentially salvageable ischaemic penumbra, and raised concentrations of glutamate which are neurotoxic.

There are few studies that have examined the effects intravenous insulin in stoke patients. The UK Glucose Insulin in Stroke Trial (GIST-UK) examined the effects of a glucose-insulin-potassium infusion to maintain euglycaemia following acute stroke. One in five of the subjects had type 2 diabetes. No effect was demonstrated on death or severe disability at 90 days. Study recruitment was much less than intended so the study was underpowered. Few subjects had a blood glucose concentration >10 mmol/l, and the difference in blood glucose concentration between the study group and control group was only 0.6 mmol/l. Further research in this area is required.

9.2.4 Secondary prevention of stroke in diabetic patients

9.2.4.1 Blood pressure

As described in Chapter 4 the treatment of hypertension is a powerful intervention for the primary prevention of strokes in people with diabetes, and this has also been demonstrated for secondary prevention. In the Perindopril Protection against Recurrent Stroke Study (PROGRESS) 6,105 patients with a previous stroke or transient ischaemic attack were allocated to placebo, or active treatment based on perindopril, with the addition of the diuretic indapamide at the discretion of the treating physicians. Overall there was a significant reduction in blood pressure and in recurrent fatal or non-fatal stroke. The reduction in blood pressure of 9/5 mmHg was slightly greater in the diabetic subgroup of 761 patients (12%). The 38% reduction in stroke was not statistically greater than the 28% reduction in patients without diabetes (Figure 9.2). There was also a significant reduction in major coronary events and heart failure in PROGRESS. Similar results were found in the Heart Outcomes Prevention Evaluation (HOPE) study with the addition of ramipril.

9.2.4.2 Statins

Studies in patients with coronary heart disease demonstrated a reduction in strokes with statin treatment. In the Heart Protection Study (HPS) overall there was a 25% reduction with simvastatin in the first event rate for stroke, with a definite reduction in ischaemic strokes and no apparent difference in haemorrhagic strokes. Simvastatin also reduced transient ischaemic attacks and the need for carotid endarterectomy or angioplasty. Analysis of patients in HPS with prior cerebrovascular disease demonstrated no apparent reduction in the stroke rate, but a significant reduction in major vascular events.

The Stroke Prevention by Aggressive Reduction in Cholesterol Levels (SPARCL) study in 4,731 patients with previous stroke or TIA has demonstrated that 80 mg of atorvastatin significantly reduced the primary endpoint of fatal or nonfatal stroke compared to placebo, and reduced the secondary outcome of major cardiovascular events. 794 patients (17%) had diabetes, but subgroup analysis was not presented.

9.2.4.3 Hyperglycaemia
The PROactive study examined the effects of pioglitazone on recurrent vascular events in 5,238 patients with type 2 diabetes and existing cardiovascular disease. 984 (19%) of the patients had previous stroke disease and on follow-up there was a highly significant 47% reduction in recurrent fatal or nonfatal stroke (Figure 9.3).

9.2.4.4 Antiplatelet drugs
Antiplatelet drugs have been proven on meta-analysis to reduce recurrent vascular events, including strokes, in diabetic patients with existing vascular disease. The optimal dose of aspirin for vascular protection in people with diabetes is till uncertain.

Meta-analysis has also demonstrated that the combination of aspirin plus dipyridamole is more effect than aspirin alone at reducing further strokes, including subgroup analysis for people with diabetes.

A recent study showed non-inferiority of clopidogrel to the combination of aspirin plus dipyridamole, but diabetes data were not reported. Another study examined the role of combined clopidogrel and aspirin in patients with previous cerebrovascular disease, and 68% of the study population had diabetes. Combined therapy produced an insignificant reduction in ischaemic stroke that was offset by a higher bleeding rate.

Thus either the combination of aspirin plus dipyridamole or clopidogrel alone should be used for secondary prevention of stroke in patients with diabetes.

9.3 **Peripheral arterial disease**

Peripheral arterial disease (PAD) is common in people with diabetes, is present in around 10% of patients at the time of diagnosis of

Figure 9.2 Effects of blood pressure lowering on the risk of stroke and other outcomes for patients with diabetes and non-diabetic subjects in the PROGRESS trial

	Events active[†] (n=3051)	Events placebo[†] (n=3054)	Favours active	Favours placebo	Hazard ratio (95% CI)	p homogeneity
STROKE						
Diabetes	48	65			0.62 (0.42–0.92)	
No diabetes	259	355			0.72 (0.61–0.84)	0.51
Ischaemic stroke						
Diabetes	42	55			0.66 (0.43–1.00)	
No diabetes	204	264			0.77 (0.64–0.92)	0.50
Large artery						
Diabetes	7	7			0.77 (0.23–2.61)	
No diabetes	25	45			0.55 (0.33–0.90)	0.62
Lacunar						
Diabetes	12	17			0.52 (0.22–1.23)	
No diabetes	52	66			0.78 (0.54–1.12)	0.41
Cardioembolic						
Diabetes	3	3			0.93 (0.19–4.6)	
No diabetes	17	23			0.75 (0.40–1.4)	0.80
Unknown type						
Diabetes	25	35			0.65 (0.38–1.13)	
No diabetes	125	149			0.84 (0.66–1.07)	0.40
Haemorrhagic stroke						
Diabetes	3	6			0.46 (0.11–1.83)	
No diabetes	34	68			0.50 (0.33–0.76)	0.90
Stroke of unknown type						
Diabetes	3	7			0.40 (0.10–1.54)	
No diabetes	39	44			0.89 (0.58–1.37)	0.44
MAJOR CHD EVENT						
Diabetes	30	21			1.31 (0.75–2.30)	
No diabetes	85	133			0.65 (0.49–0.86)	0.03
HEART FAILURE						
Diabetes	25	33			0.67 (0.40–1.15)	
No diabetes	88	118			0.74 (0.56–0.98)	0.76
MAJOR VASCULAR EVENTS						
Diabetes	82	91			0.79 (0.58–1.07)	
No diabetes	376	513			0.72 (0.63–0.82)	0.56
COGNITION						
Dementia[†]						
Diabetes	24	25			0.84 (0.47–1.53)	
No diabetes	169	192			0.89 (0.72–1.10)	0.88
Cognitive decline[†]						
Diabetes	48	41			1.10 (0.71–1.72)	
No diabetes	228	293			0.76 (0.64–0.92)	0.14

0.5   1.0   2.0
Hazard ratio & 95% CI

type 2 diabetes, and will develop in up to 45% of patients on long-term follow up. Diabetes greatly increases the risk of claudication, and the risk of non-traumatic lower limb amputation is increased between ten and sixteen-fold in diabetes. Morbidity and mortality from PAD is increased in diabetes, the disease is more progressive, and the response to revascularization is less successful than in non-diabetic subjects. Risk factors for the development of PAD and for amputation are shown in Box 9.1. Diabetes tends to cause more diffuse and distal disease, and there is more vascular calcification. The clinical presentation of PAD in diabetes is shown in Table 9.1.

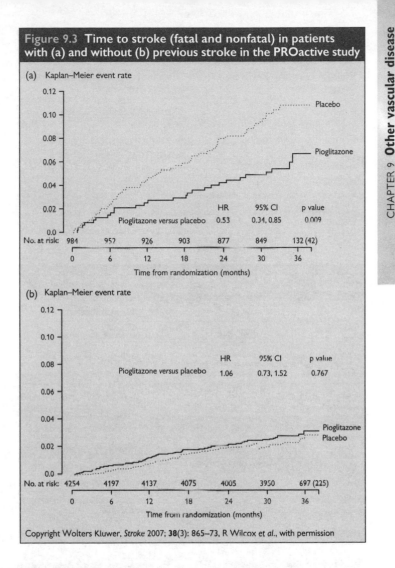

Figure 9.3 Time to stroke (fatal and nonfatal) in patients with (a) and without (b) previous stroke in the PROactive study

(a) Kaplan–Meier event rate

Pioglitazone versus placebo | HR 0.53 | 95% CI 0.34, 0.85 | p value 0.009

(b) Kaplan–Meier event rate

Pioglitazone versus placebo | HR 1.06 | 95% CI 0.73, 1.52 | p value 0.767

Copyright Wolters Kluwer, *Stroke* 2007; **38**(3): 865–73, R Wilcox et al., with permission

9.4 **Treatment of PAD in diabetes**

Revascularization with either angioplasty or arterial bypass surgery may help to heal leg ulcers, and graft survival rate is the same as in non-diabetic subjects. The medical management of PAD in diabetes comprises an intensive multi-risk factor intervention, although the specific evidence for benefit for patients with PAD is slight, and treatment has been extrapolated from other forms of vascular disease (Table 9.2).

Box 9.1 Risk factors for PAD and for amputation in patients with diabetes

Risk factors for PAD in diabetes	Risk factors for amputation in diabetes
<ul><li>age</li><li>high HbA1c</li><li>raised systolic blood pressure</li><li>low HDL cholesterol</li><li>smoking</li><li>other cardiovascular disease</li><li>retinopathy</li><li>sensory neuropathy</li></ul>	<ul><li>poor glycaemic control</li><li>age</li><li>ethnicity, especially Blacks</li><li>smoking</li></ul>

Table 9.1 Comparisons of peripheral arterial disease (PAD) in diabetic and non-diabetic subjects

	Diabetic	Non-diabetic
Prevalence	~ higher	~ lower
Age	Younger	Older
Male: Female	M=F	M > F
Lower extremities affected	Both	Unilateral
Occlusion	Multi-segmental, distal	Single segment, proximal
Vessels involved	Tibials, peroneals	Aortic, iliac, femoral
Vessels adjacent to occlusion	Affected	Not affected
Collaterals	Affected	Not affected

Table 9.2 Multi-factorial management of peripheral arterial disease (PAD) in diabetes

Risk factor	Intervention
Smoking	Smoking cessation
Thrombotic tendency	Aspirin or clopidogrel
Hyperglycaemia	Anti-diabetic drugs
Dyslipidaemia	Statins
Hypertension	Anti-hypertensive drugs
'At-risk foot'	Education on footcare, regular podiatry

9.4.1 **Smoking cessation**

Smoking increases the risk of developing PAD and reduces patency rates and survival following revascularization procedures. There is little information on the effects of smoking cessation in diabetes, and the approach is similar to non-diabetic subjects with behavioural support supplemented by the use of nicotine replacement therapy or varenicline.

9.4.2 **Antiplatelet therapy**

In non-diabetic subjects antiplatelet therapy delays the progression of established PAD, but again specific data in diabetes is lacking. As for other clinical situations the optimal dose of aspirin for patients with diabetes has not been established. In the Clopidogrel versus Aspirin in Patients at Risk of Ischaemic Events (CAPRIE) study clopidogrel was more effective than aspirin in reducing myocardial infarctions and vascular deaths for patients with PAD, but data for diabetic patients with PAD was not provided.

9.4.3 **Glycaemic control**

In the UKPDS there was a trend towards a reduction in amputations and deaths from PAD in the tight control group, but this did not reach statistical significance. In the DCCT there was an insignificant reduction major lower limb complications. In the EDIC follow-up reduced peripheral arterial calcification was observed in patients who had previously been intensively treated.

9.4.4 **Dyslipidaemia**

In HPS patients with baseline peripheral arterial disease had a significant reduction in vascular events with simvastatin, and in patients with diabetes there was a significant reduction in a composite of peripheral vascular complications, which included any peripheral arterial surgery, peripheral angioplasty, leg amputation or leg ulcer.

9.4.5 **Hypertension**

Hypertension is a risk factor for peripheral arterial disease, but the evidence that lowering blood pressure reduces peripheral arterial events is limited. In the HOPE study (not strictly speaking a blood pressure study) subjects with peripheral arterial disease at baseline had a highly significant reduction in the primary composite endpoint with ramipril. Overall ramipril-treated subjects had less coronary and lower extremity revascularization procedures. There should be close monitoring of renal function when ACE inhibitors are started in diabetic patients with PAD in case there is concomitant renal artery stenosis (see Section 9.6).

9.5 **Erectile dysfunction**

9.5.1 **Erectile dysfunction, diabetes and cardiovascular disease**

The process of penile erection is a physiological neurovascular event resulting from smooth muscle relaxation, triggered and modified by neural, endocrine and psychological components. Erectile dysfunction (ED) can be defined as the consistent or recurrent inability of a man to attain and/or maintain a penile erection sufficient for sexual performance. The association between diabetes and erectile dysfunction is well established, ED is three times more common in men with diabetes, and at least 50% of men with diabetes will suffer from ED at some time. The pathophysiology of erectile dysfunction is multifactorial and includes endothelial and smooth muscle dysfunction and autonomic neuropathy in addition to psychological and interpersonal issues.

Risk factors for the development of ED in diabetes are shown in Box 9.2. It can be seen that several risk factors for ED are also risk factors for cardiovascular disease. The link between ED and cardiovascular risk factors may be endothelial dysfunction of tissue within the corpus cavernosum. In one study ED was a marker for future cardiovascular events with a risk that was equivalent to smoking or a family history of myocardial infarction. In diabetic men ED can be associated with symptomatic coronary artery disease or silent myocardial ischaemia, and some authorities recommend screening for silent coronary disease in diabetic men who present with ED. There are also several cardiovascular medications that may be associated with an increased risk of ED (Box 9.3).

9.5.2 **Treatment considerations**

Oral treatments for ED are phosphodiesterase type-5 (PDE5) inhibitors, which inhibit the breakdown of cyclic GMP, and there are three available for clinical use (sildenafil, tadalafil, vardenafil). Interestingly,

Box 9.2 Risk factors for erectile dysfunction in diabetes	
Risk factors	**Protective factors**
• increasing age • smoking • longer duration of diabetes • poor metabolic control • untreated hypertension • neuropathy • microalbuminuria • macroalbuminuria • retinopathy • cardiovascular disease	• increased physical activity • moderate alcohol consumption

---

Box 9.3 Drugs possibly associated with an increased risk of erectile dysfunction

Antihypertensive drugs

- thiazide diuretcs
- beta-blockers
- central sympatholytics (methyldopa, clonidine)
- spironolactone
- calcium-channel blockers?
- ACE inhibitors?

Other cardiovascular medications

- statins
- fibrates
- digoxin

---

the effect of sildenafil on erectile function was first noticed when it was being investigated as a possible treatment for angina. PDE5 inhibitors are contraindicated in patients receiving nitrates, as the combination can cause a precipitous drop in blood pressure and coronary perfusion, and in particular decreases in coronary flow rate in blood vessels with a critical coronary stenosis. Nicorandil acts as a nitric oxide donor and is also contraindicated. An expert's consensus prepared by the American Heart Association has described several relative contraindications to the use of PDE5 inhibitors in patients with cardiovascular disease (Box 9.4).

9.6 **Renovascular disease**

Renal artery stenosis is common in type 2 diabetes and contributes to renal impairment and hypertension. In these patients the use of

---

Box 9.4 Contraindications to PDE5 inhibitors

Absolute

- nitrate therapy
- nicorandil therapy

Relative

- active coronary insufficiency
- heart failure with low blood pressure
- patients with combination therapies involving three or four drugs for hypertension
- patients taking anti-arrhythmic drugs with the exception of beta-blockers

---

ACE inhibitors or angiotensin-II receptor blockers can lead to acute renal failure, especially if renal artery stenosis affects both kidneys, or a single functioning kidney. Diabetic patients with unexplained progressive renal impairment, especially in the absence of proteinuria or retinopathy, with hypertension that is poorly controlled despite the use of multiple antihypertensive drugs, or with 'flash' pulmonary oedema should be investigated for possible renal artery stenosis. Ultrasonography is the first line method of imaging, but a normal renal ultrasound does not exclude possible renal artery stenosis. Magnetic resonance angiography and CT angiography are the preferred non-invasive imaging modalities, and digital subtraction angiography should be reserved for patients in whom intervention is being considered, or if non-invasive imaging is inconclusive. Revascularization either by angioplasty and stenting or direct surgical revascularization may stabilize renal function bur rarely improves blood pressure management, and appears to be of little long-term benefit.

9.7 **Other vascular disease in diabetes**

Atheroma affecting other vascular beds such as the gastrointestinal tract also seem to be more common in diabetes, and can be difficult to diagnose.

References

Berthet K, Neal BC, Chalmers JP, et al. on behalf of the PROGRESS Collaborative Group. (2004) Reductions in the risks of recurrent stroke in patients with and without diabetes: the PROGRESS trial. *Blood Pressrue* **13**: 7–13.

Bhasin S, Enzlin P, Coviello A, Basson R (2007) Sexual dysfunction in men and women with endocrine disorders. *Lancet* **369**: 597–611.

Gray CS, Hildreth AJ, Sandercock PA, et al. for the GIST Trialists Collaboration. (2007) Glucose-potassium-insulin infusions in the management of post-stroke hyperglycaemia: the UK Glucose Insulin in Stroke Trial (GIST-UK). *Lancet Neurology* **6**: 397–406.

Krempf M, Parhofer KG, Steg G, et al. (2010) Cardiovascular event rates in diabetic and nondiabetic individuals with and without atherothrombosis (from the Reduction of Atherothrobosis for Continued health [REACH] Registry). *American Journal of Cardiology* **105**: 667–71.

Idris I, Donnelly R (2007) Diabetes and peripheral arterial disease. In M Fisher and JJ McMurray, eds *Diabetic cardiology*, pp. 199–222, John Wiley & Sons, Ltd, Chichester, UK.

Stroke Prevention by Aggressive Reduction in Cholesterol Levels (SPARCL) Investigators (2006) High-dose atorvastatin after stroke or transient ischemic attack. *New England Journal of Medicine* **355**: 549–59.

Wilcox R, Bousser MG, Betteridge DJ, *et al.* for the PROactive Investigators. (2007). Effects of pioglitazone in patients with type 2 diabetes with or without previous stroke: results from PROactive (PROspective pioglitAzone Clinical Trial in macroVascular Events 04). *Stroke* **38**: 865–73.

Chapter 10

Diabetic nephropathy

Miles Fisher

Key points

- Diabetic nephropathy develops in 40% of patients with type 1 diabetes and 30% of patients with type 2 diabetes
- Microalbuminuria is a marker of patients who will progress to overt diabetic nephropathy, and indicates a poor cardiovascular prognosis
- A multi-risk factor intervention for patients with type 2 diabetes and microalbuminuria reduces renal and cardiovascular outcomes
- In type 1 diabetes the aggressive treatment of hypertension in patients with overt nephropathy with therapy based on ACE inhibitors reduces cardiovascular and renal outcomes
- In type 2 diabetes the aggressive treatment of hypertension in patients with overt nephropathy with therapy based on ACE inhibitors or angiotensin-II receptor antagonists reduces renal outcomes, but reductions in cardiovascular events are less impressive.

10.1 Diabetic nephropathy

10.1.1 Epidemiology of diabetic nephropathy

Diabetic nephropathy is one of the principal causes of chronic kidney disease in patients starting renal replacement therapy. It is associated with a high cardiovascular mortality, and many patients with diabetic nephropathy will die from cardiovascular causes before renal function has decreased to the point where renal replacement therapy is required. The earliest stage of nephropathy is microalbuminuria, which predicts the later development of macroalbuminuria, also termed 'overt nephropathy', or 'clinical nephropathy'. Microalbuminuria is also a strong predictor of cardiovascular events in patients with type 1 and type 2 diabetes.

Ten per cent of patients with type 1 diabetes will develop microalbuminuria after 7 years, and on long-term follow-up 40% will develop macroalbuminuria if untreated. In patients with type 2 diabetes a quarter will have microalbuminuria after 10 years. The prevalence of macroalbuminuria varies from 5–20% because of the increased cardiovascular mortality, but because of the much greater prevalence of type 2 diabetes this is still the most common type of diabetes in patients requiring renal replacement therapy.

10.1.2 Nephropathy and cardiovascular risk

The poor prognosis of patients with microalbuminuria may be a reflection of generalised endothelial dysfunction. Slight reductions in glomerular filtration rate also significantly increase cardiovascular risk. Further reduction in renal function leads to hypertension, left ventricular hypertrophy, accelerated coronary heart disease, and a dilated cardiomyopathy, which manifest clinically as angina, myocardial infarction, chronic heart failure and premature death. There is also a close association between diabetic renal failure, peripheral vascular disease, foot ulcers, gangrene, and amputations.

10.2 Microalbuminurua

10.2.1 Microalbuminuria and type 1 diabetes

In patients with type 1 diabetes regression of microalbuminuria is relatively common, and regression is associated with shorter duration of diabetes, lower systolic blood pressure, tighter control of glycaemia, and lower concentrations of cholesterol and triglycerides. Once microalbuminuria is established, the aggressive treatment of glycaemia and of hypertension and reduces the progression from microalbuminuria to overt nephropathy, and ACE inhibitors have effects that are partly independent of blood pressure lowering. ACE inhibitors can slow the progression of renal disease in patients with type 1 diabetes who are normotensive.

10.2.2 ACE inhibitors, microalbuminuria, and type 2 diabetes

Several small studies have shown beneficial effects of ACE inhibitors on microalbuminuria in patients with type 2 diabetes. In addition, trandolapril has been shown to prevent the development of microalbuminuria in patients with type 2 diabetes. The large Microalbuminuria, Cardiovascular and Renal Outcomes in the Heart Outcomes Prevention Evaluation (MICRO-HOPE)

Table 10.1 Results from the MICRO-HOPE study	
Cardiovascular	**Renal**
Reduced myocardial infarction	Reduced overt nephropathy
Reduced strokes	Reduced mean albumin:creatinine ratio
Reduced cardiovascular deaths	Reduced new microalbuminuria (not significant)
Reduced total mortality	
Reduced revascularizations	

diabetes sub study from the Heart Outcomes Prevention Evaluation (HOPE study) examined the effects of ramipril on cardiovascular and renal outcomes in people who mostly had type 2 diabetes. The primary endpoint of cardiovascular death, myocardial infarction and strokes was significantly reduced with ramipril. Renal endpoints were included in secondary outcomes, but unfortunately sampling for microalbuminuria and proteinuria was performed infrequently throughout the study. There was a significant reduction in the progression of microalbuminuria with ramipril, and a significant reduction in the development of overt nephropathy (Table 10.1).

The Diabetes, Hypertension, cardiovascular events, and Ramipril (DIABHYCAR) study examined the effects of low dose ramipril (1.25 mg) on cardiovascular and renal outcomes in patients with type 2 diabetes and raised excretion of urinary albumin. Ramipril lowered blood pressure slightly, and favoured regression from microalbuminuria to normal, but had no effect on a composite outcome of cardiovascular death, non-fatal myocardial infarction, stroke, heart failure hospitalization, or end stage renal failure, or on any components of the endpoint.

This study suggests that low dose ACE inhibition may reduce albumin excretion, but not cardiovascular or renal outcomes which require full-dose ACE inhibition.

10.2.3 Angiotensin-II receptor antagonists, microalbuminuria, and type 2 diabetes

Angiotensin-II receptor antagonists (ARAs), have been studied in patients with type 2 diabetes. The Irbesartan in Patients with Type 2 Diabetes and Microalbuminuria Study (IRMA-2) compared irbesartan in two doses (150 mg, 300 mg) with placebo in patients with hypertension and microalbuminuria. Irbesartan reduced the progression to persistent albuminuria and increase regression to normal albumin excretion. A similar, shorter study with valsartan

Box 10.1 Results from the IRMA-2 study

Principal results

- In hypertensive patients with type 2 diabetes and microalbuminuria irbesartan reduced the progression to persistent albuminuria. There was a slightly greater reduction in systolic blood pressure with irbesartan compared to the placebo group.

Other cardiovascular results

- 24-hour ambulatory blood pressure monitoring in a subpopulation of IRMA2 showed that irbesartan was renoprotective independently of beneficial effects in lowering 24 hour blood pressure.

- Irbesartan reduced markers of low-grade inflammation, including high-sensitivity C-reactive protein and fibrinogen, and attenuated the increase in interleukin-6 (IL-6). Changes in IL-6 were associated with changes in albumin excretion, and the reduction in low-grade inflammation with irbesartan may have reduced the risk of microvascular and macrovascular disease.

- One month after withdrawal of treatment blood pressure rose in the patients who received irbesartan, but urinary albumin excretion was persistently reduced in the patients who had received irbesartan 300 mg after withdrawal of therapy.

(Microalbuminuria Reduction with Valsartan, MARVAL) showed similar benefits compared to amlodipine, indicating that some of the reduction in albumin excretion was related to blood pressure reductions and some to the specific agent. There have been a few other publications from the IRMA-2 study that have given useful information about microalbuminuria and type 2 diabetes (Box 10.1). In the IRMA-2 study mean blood pressure with 300 mg irbesartan was 141/83 mmHg.

The Diabetics Exposed to Telmisartan and Enalapril (DETAIL) study compared the effects of the ARA telmisartan with the ACE inhibitor enalapril in a small group of patients with type 2 diabetes and early nephropathy. 80% had microalbuminuria, and half had a history of cardiovascular disease. The primary endpoint was the change in the glomerular filtration rate, and the effects of the two drugs were not significantly different. There was no difference in the rates of end-stage renal disease or cardiovascular events, which were secondary end points. Similar results were found in a smaller, shorter study which found equal reductions in blood pressure, urinary albumin excretion, and rate of decline in glomerular filtration rate comparing losartan and enalapril in hypertensive type 2 diabetic patients with early nephropathy.

Several short-term studies have examined the effects of combining ACE inhibitors and ARAs in diabetic patients with microalbuminuria. The combination leads to greater reductions in blood pressure and microalbuminuria than a single drug, but long term studies examining the effects of the combination on the progression to overt nephropathy in diabetes, and on cardiovascular outcomes, are awaited.

10.2.4 **Other drugs**

Aliskiren is a novel renin inhibitor which blocks the renin-angiotensin system and lowers blood pressure. A short study in type 2 diabetes showed a reduction in albumin excretion in patients with type 2 diabetes and microalbuminuria, and long-term studies on the progression of nephropathy and on cardiovascular outcomes are under way.

10.2.5 **Multi-factorial risk intervention for microalbuminuria**

The Steno-2 study was a comparison of targeted, intensified, multi-factorial intervention with conventional treatment in a small group of patients with type 2 diabetes and microalbuminuria. Interventions in the intensive therapy group comprised:

- advice on diet, exercise, and smoking cessation
- intensive blood glucose control with a target HbA1c below 6.5%
- the use of an ACE inhibitor irrespective of blood pressure
- aggressive treatment of hypertension
- statins for raised cholesterol and fibrates for raised triglycerides
- aspirin
- vitamin and mineral supplementation.

More patients in the intensive group reached targets for blood pressure, lipids and HbA1c, and the blood glucose targets were the hardest to achieve. Patients receiving intensive therapy had a significantly lower risk of cardiovascular disease, nephropathy, retinopathy, and autonomic neuropathy, with a 50% reduction in events over eight years (Figure 10.1) When specific cardiovascular events were examined the reduction in strokes was statistically significant, but the reductions in myocardial infarction and coronary interventions (PCI or CABG) did not reach individual statistical significance (Figure 10.2). Post trial monitoring out to 13 years showed a reduction in total and cardiovascular mortality (Figure 10.3).

10.2.6 **Antioxidants**

In the Steno-2 study a multivitamin preparation was included as antioxidant treatment. Many large, multi-centre studies, including large numbers of patients with type 2 diabetes, have examined the possible reduction in cardiac events with antioxidant therapy, and these have been negative. A large study examining the possible benefits

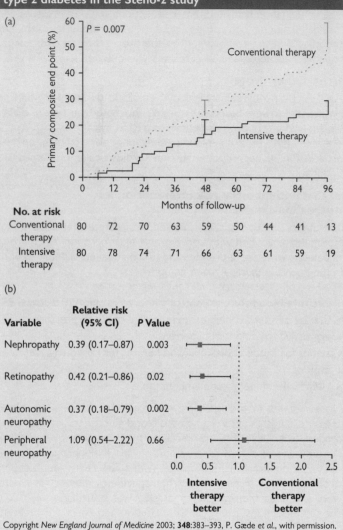

Figure 10.1 Effects of intensive multifactorial intervention in type 2 diabetes in the Steno-2 study

Copyright *New England Journal of Medicine* 2003; **348**:383–393, P. Gæde *et al.*, with permission.

of aspirin and/or multivitamins in patients with type 2 diabetes is currently being run in the UK.

10.3 **Macroalbuminuria treatments**

A small but detailed study from the Steno Hospital, Denmark, that was performed in the 1980s demonstrated that aggressive

Figure 10.2 Effects of intensive multifactorial intervention in type 2 diabetes on cardiovascular events in the Steno-2 study A: Distribution of the total number of cardiovascular events in the intensive therapy group in the Steno-2 Study (light purple) and the conventional therapy group (purple). **B:** Kaplan-Meier estimates of time to first stroke in the intensive therapy and conventional therapy group. HR, hazard ratio. **C:** Kaplan-Meier estimates of time to first percutaneous intervention (PCI) or coronary bypass graft (CABG) in the intensive therapy and conventional therapy group. **D:** Kaplan-Meier estimates of time to first myocardial infarction in the intensive therapy and conventional therapy group

Copyright American Diabetes Association, *Diabetes* 2004 vol. **53** (3): S39–S47, P. Gæde *et al.*, with permission

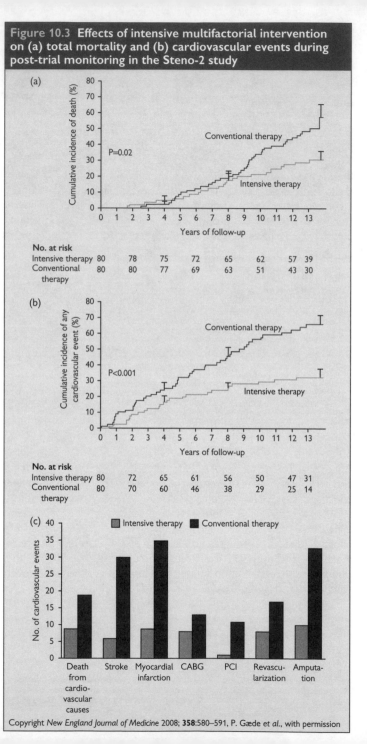

Figure 10.3 **Effects of intensive multifactorial intervention on (a) total mortality and (b) cardiovascular events during post-trial monitoring in the Steno-2 study**

Copyright *New England Journal of Medicine* 2008; **358**:580–591, P. Gæde et al., with permission antihypertensive treatment, based on treatment with metoprolol, hydralazine and furosemide, reduced albuminuria and the decline in glomerular filtration rate in patients with type 1 diabetes and overt nephropathy.

10.3.1 **ACE inhibitors and type 1 diabetes**

A larger, multicentre study performed by the Collaborative Study Group compared the ACE inhibitor captopril with placebo in 409 patients with type 1 diabetes and diabetic nephropathy. Target blood pressure goals were set for all subjects. Captopril reduced the primary end point which was a doubling of the baseline serum creatinine concentration. There was also a significant reduction in a combined end point of death, dialysis and transplantation. There were 8 deaths in the captopril group and 11 in the placebo group, but individual causes of death were not reported.

10.3.2 **Angiotensin-II receptor antagonists and type 2 diabetes**

There are several small studies showing that ACE inhibitors reduce proteinuria and the decline in glomerular filtration rate in patients with type 2 diabetes and overt nephropathy, but none of these studies was statistically powered to look at the progression to end-stage renal replacement or cardiovascular outcomes. Two large multicentre studies were performed using the ARBs losartan and irbesartan in patients with type 2 diabetes and overt nephropathy, and there was criticism of the ethics of the study design as comparisons were made with placebo or amlodipine, and not with ACE inhibitors which were deemed to be the best treatment at the time the studies were designed.

In the Reduction of Endpoints in NIDDM with the Angiotensin II Antagonist Losartan (RENAAL) study losartan reduced the primary end point which was a composite of doubling of base-line creatinine concentration, end-stage renal disease or death. When the components of the composite were examined, losartan reduced the doubling or serum creatinine and end-stage renal disease, but had no effect on deaths. There was no effect on a secondary composite of morbidity and mortality from cardiovascular causes, although the rate of first hospitalisation for heart failure was significantly lower with losartan (Figure 10.4).

There have been multiple other publications from the RENAAL study, including several that have given useful information about cardiovascular risk and nephropathy in type 2 diabetes (Box 10.2).

In the Irbesartan Diabetic Nephropathy Trial (IDNT) irbesartan reduced the same primary end point of a doubling of the baseline serum creatinine concentration, end-stage renal disease or death compared to placebo and amlodipine, indicating that protection was independent of reductions in blood pressure. There was no

Figure 10.4 Reduction in heart failure hospitalizations with losartan in the RENAAL study

Risk reduction, 32%
P = 0.005

First hospitalization for heart failure (%)

Placebo

Losartan

Months of study

No. at risk				
Placebo	762	685	616	375	53
Losartan	751	701	637	388	74

Copyright *New England Journal of Medicine* 2001; **345**:861–869, B. Brenenr et al., with permission

---

Box 10.2 Results from the RENAAL study

Principal results

- In patients with type 2 diabetes and overt nephropathy losartan reduced the primary outcome which was a composite of doubling of base-line creatinine, end-stage renal disease, or death.

Other important results

- Elderly patients (>65 years) had the same level of benefit and risks from treatment with losartan.
- Baseline systolic blood pressure was a stronger predictor than diastolic blood pressure of renal outcomes and death.
- Baseline total and LDL cholesterol and triglyceride levels were associated with increased risk of developing the primary composite end point, and were not adversely affected by losartan.
- ECG criteria of baseline left ventricular hypertrophy was associated with a significantly increased risk of cardiovascular events and the progression of kidney disease.
- Among all the baseline risk markers, albuminuria was the strongest predictor of cardiovascular outcomes, and reducing albuminuria in the first six months appeared to afford cardiovascular protection.

Box 10.3 Results from the IDNT study

Principal results

- Irbesartan was effective in protecting against the progression of nephropathy in type 2 diabetes, independently of reductions in blood pressure.

Other important results

- Further analysis of the cardiovascular composite showed a lower incidence of congestive cardiac failure with irbesartan compared with placebo, a trend towards a decrease in strokes in patients receiving amlodipine, and a significantly lower rate of myocardial infarction with amlodipine compared with placebo.
- Clinically unrecognized myocardial infarction that was detected by the development of Q waves on the electrocardiogram accounted for 14% of all non-fatal myocardial infarctions.
- The degree of albuminuria at baseline and lower serum albumin levels provided additional prognostic information about the risk of cardiovascular events in addition to traditional coronary risk factors.
- An achieved systolic blood pressure approaching 120 mmHg and diastolic blood pressure of 85 mmHg were associated with the best protection against cardiovascular events. A blood pressure below 120/85 mmHg was associated with an increase in cardiovascular events.

significant effect on death as a component of the primary endpoint, or in a secondary cardiovascular composite end point, although the rate of hospitalization for heart failure was lower with irbesartan than placebo.

There have been several other publications from the IDNT study that have given useful information about cardiovascular risk and diabetic nephropathy in type 2 diabetes (Box 10.3).

10.3 Systematic reviews and meta-analysis

As mentioned above there are very few studies comparing ACE inhibitors versus Angiotensin-II receptor antagonists in patients with diabetic nephropathy. In an attempt to determine which class of drug might lead to better outcomes systematic reviews have been performed of renal and cardiovascular outcomes, and the results of these have been controversial. One systematic review concluded that there were survival benefits of ACE inhibitors for patients with diabetic nephropathy, with a reduction in all cause mortality compared with placebo. Much of this evidence came from the Collaborative Study Group study of captopril in type 1 diabetes and from the MICRO-HOPE study.

By contrast, ARAs did not have any effect on all cause mortality, and much of this data came from the IRMA-2, IDNT, and RENAAL studies. A possible biological rationale for the benefit of ACE inhibitors but not of ARAs could be the accumulation of bradykinin with ACE inhibitors (see also Chapter 4). In a similar meta-analysis which included data from LIFE, IDNT, and RENAAL studies no effect was seen on total mortality, or cardiovascular morbidity and mortality.

10.4 **Other drugs to reduce cardiovascular risk**

Other than treating blood pressure with drugs that block the rennin-angiotensin system there is little evidence for benefit of other interventions in people with established nephropathy. Anaemia is more common in diabetic kidney disease than other forms of kidney disease, can occur when renal function is only moderately impaired, and adversely affects the cardiovascular prognosis. There is a continuing debate as to what is the optimal target haemoglobin for therapy with erythropoetin or analogues in renal patients, and there are several ongoing cardiovascular endpoint studies that include many patients with diabetes. In the Trial to Reduce Cardiovascular Events with Aranesp Therapy (TREAT) trial the use of darbepoetin alfa in patients with diabetes, chronic kidney disease and aneamia did not reduce cardiovascular events and in fact was associated with an increased risk of stroke.

Statins have been examined in patients with renal failure, and the results have been negative. One study that examined the possible benefits of fluvastatin in patients with renal failure from multiple causes including diabetic nephropathy was negative. Another study examined the possible effects of atorvastatin in diabetic patients on haemodialysis and was also negative. A recent trial of simvastatin plus ezetimibe in patients with chronic kidney disease demonstrated reductions in cardiovascular events. One quarter of the subjects had diabetes. The lack of a reduction in cardiovascular endpoints with statins (and angiotensin-II receptor blockers) may partly be explained by advanced nature of the atherosclerosis in these patients.

10.5 **Conclusions**

Diabetic nephropathy is associated with a high cardiovascular mortality which worsens with increasing albumin excretion and deterioration in glomerular function. Aggressive treatment of blood pressure with drugs that block the renin-angiotensin system delays the deterioration in renal function and the need for end-stage renal replacement therapy. The evidence for reductions in cardiovascular events is less impressive, and is mostly from the use of ACE inhibitors.

References

Brenner BM, Cooper ME, de Zeeuw D, et al. for the RENAAL Study Investigators (2001) Effects of losartan on renal and cardiovascular outcomes in patients with type 2 diabetes and nephropathy. New England Journal of Medicine 345: 861–9.

Gaede P, Vedel P, Larsen N, Jensen GVH, Parving HH, and Pedersen O (2003) Multifactorial intervention and cardiovascular disease in patients with type 2 diabetes. New England Journal of Medicine 348: 383–93.

Gaede P, Lund-Andersen H, Parving H-H, Pedersen O (2008) Effect of a multifactorial intervention on mortality in type 2 diabetes. New England Journal of Medicine 358: 580–91.

Heart Outcomes and Prevention Evaluation (HOPE) Study Investigators (2000) Effects of ramipril on cardiovascular and microvascular outcomes in people with diabetes mellitus: results of the HOPE study and MICRO-HOPE substudy. Lancet 355: 253–9.

Lewis EJ, Hunsicker LG, Bain RP and Rohde RD (1993) The effect of angiotensin-converting-enzyme inhibition on diabetic nephropathy. The Collaborative Study Group. New England Journal of Medicine 329: 1456–62.

Lewis EJ, Hunsicker LG, Clarke WR, et al. for the Collaborative Study Group (2001) Renoprotective effect of the angiotensin-receptor antagonist irbesartan in patients with nephropathy due to type 2 diabetes. New England Journal of Medicine 345: 851–60.

Parving H-H, Lehnert H, Brochner-Mortensen J, et al. for the Irbesartan in Patients with Type 2 Diabetes and Microalbuminuria Study Group. (2001) The effect of irbesartan on the development of diabetic nephropathy in patients with type 2 diabetes. New England Journal of Medicine 345: 870–8

Parving H-H, Persson F, Lewis JB, Lewis EK, Hollenberg NK for the AVOID Study Investigators (2008) Aliskiren combined with losartan in type 2 diabetes and nephropathy. New England Journal of Medicine 358: 2433–46.

Chapter 11

Diabetic autonomic neuropathy and sudden death in diabetes

Miles Fisher

Key points

- Symptomatic diabetic autonomic neuropathy is uncommon in type 1 diabetes, but may cause postural hypotension and may limit exercise tolerance
- Symptomatic autonomic neuropathy carries a poor prognosis and sudden cardio-respiratory arrest is described
- Asymptomatic abnormalities of cardiac autonomic function are common in patients with type 1 diabetes and type 2 diabetes
- A syndrome of 'dead in bed' is described in type 1 diabetes in patients with longstanding diabetes, which may be caused by nocturnal hypoglycaemia in patients with abnormal autonomic function provoking serious arrhythmias.

129

11.1 Clinical description of diabetic autonomic neuropathy

Diabetes is the most common cause of autonomic neuropathy in developed countries. Symptomatic autonomic neuropathy is a late complication of diabetes. It is typically seen in patients that also have a distal sensorimotor polyneuropathy. The autonomic nervous system controls the electrical and contractile activity of the heart through an interaction of sympathetic and parasympathetic fibres. 'Cardiac autonomic neuropathy' indicates dysfunction of the autonomic nerves to and from the heart and 'cardiovascular autonomic neuropathy' includes damage to the fibres enervating the heart and

Box 11.1 Risk factors for diabetic cardiovascular autonomic neuropathy

- age
- duration of diabetes
- poor glycaemic control
- hypertension
- dyslipdaemia
- obesity
- lack of physical fitness
- smoking
- diabetic nephropathy
- retinopathy
- distal symmetrical polyneuropathy ('peripheral neuropathy')

blood vessels, resulting in abnormalities of heart rate and blood pressure control. Patients with symptomatic autonomic neuropathy have a poor prognosis and the cause of death is often cardio-respiratory arrest or sudden death.

11.1.1 **Epidemiology and aetiology**

Testing for autonomic neuropathy is not done routinely so there is little information about the epidemiology of diabetic autonomic neuropathy. Studies have tended to be cross-sectional rather than prospective, have included short follow-up periods, and different methods of assessment have been used. Asymptomatic abnormalities are common when testing autonomic cardiovascular reflexes in diabetes, and may be found in 40% of patients. Risk factors for cardiovascular autonomic neuropathy are described in Box 11.1 Although hyperglycaemia and duration of diabetes have major roles, insulin resistance and hyperinsulinaemia also play a part. In the DCCT intensive glycaemic control reduced the development of diabetic autonomic neuropathy, and benefits persisted in the EDIC follow-up.

11.2 **Symptomatic cardiovascular autonomic neuropathy**

11.2.1 **Resting tachycardia and palpitations**

The resting heart rate is higher in diabetic populations compared with non-diabetic populations, reflecting early parasympathetic neuropathy, although this is still usually within the normal range of <100 beats per minute. As the parasympathetic vagal neuropathy worsens a true resting tachycardia (>100 beats per minute.) develops because of unopposed sympathetic stimulation. This may be noticed by the patient and may occasionally give a sensation of palpitations. With more profound sympathetic neuropathy the heart rate lowers again, and in severe neuropathy the heart rate is fixed and does not respond to exercise or other stimuli.

11.2.2 **Postural hypotension**

Postural, or 'orthostatic' hypotension is a fall in blood pressure in response to a change from lying to standing. It occurs because of an efferent sympathetic vasomotor denervation with reduced vasoconstriction of splanchnic and other vascular beds. It can cause symptoms of weakness, dizziness, faintness, visual upset, pre-syncope or syncope. By contrast, some diabetic patients may have profound drops in systolic blood pressure on standing that are completely asymptomatic.

Postural hypotension can be a difficult to treat, and simple measures such as fluid repletion and salt supplementation or wearing support stockings are often ineffective. Fludrocortisone may relieve symptoms by expanding plasma volume, and a sympathomimetic agent such as midodrine can be added if symptoms persist (Figure 11.1).

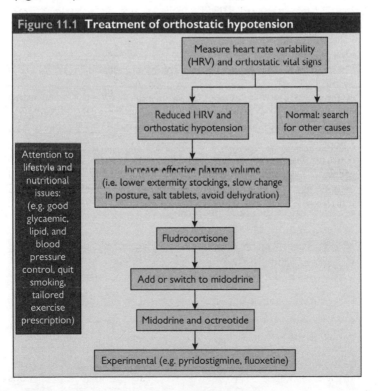

Figure 11.1 Treatment of orthostatic hypotension

Measure heart rate variability (HRV) and orthostatic vital signs

Reduced HRV and orthostatic hypotension

Normal: search for other causes

Attention to lifestyle and nutritional issues: (e.g. good glycaemic, lipid, and blood pressure control, quit smoking, tailored exercise prescription)

Increase effective plasma volume (i.e. lower extermity stockings, slow change in posture, salt tablets, avoid dehydration)

Fludrocortisone

Add or switch to midodrine

Midodrine and octreotide

Experimental (e.g. pyridostigmine, fluoxetine)

11.2.3 **Reduced exercise capacity**

The physiological response to exercise includes reduction in parasympathetic neural tone and activation of the sympathetic nervous system, including direct effects via sympathetic stimulation and indirect effects secondary to the release of epinephrine from the adrenal medulla. This enhances cardiac output and increases blood flow to skeletal muscle. These mechanisms can be affected by autonomic neuropathy, reducing the heart and blood pressure responses to exercise, with a lesser increase in cardiac output, and a reduced exercise tolerance which is noticed by the patients as early fatigue. Reduced ejection fraction, systolic dysfunction and decreased diastolic filling also limit exercise tolerance.

11.2.4 **Silent myocardial ischaemia**

Strictly speaking this is the absence of a symptom, related to neuropathy of the afferent pain fibres which are carried from the heart in the vagus nerve. Silent myocardial ischaemia is more common in people with diabetes, and is partly explained by a cardiovascular autonomic neuropathy (see also Chapter 5). As pain is a symptom that leads the patient to attend a doctor and undergo further investigation, the presence of silent or atypical ischaemia delays investigation and may partly explain the increase in sudden fatalities from acute myocardial infarction in diabetes.

11.3 **Assessment of autonomic function**

Simple assessment of autonomic function can be performed using a battery of non-invasive cardiovascular reflex tests (Box 11.2). These involve the measurement of changes in heart rate and blood

---

Box 11.2 Tests of cardiovascular autonomic function in diabetes

Cardiovascular autonomic reflex tests
- Heart rate response to deep breathing
- Heart rate response to standing
- Heart rate response to the Valsalva manoeuvre
- Systolic blood pressure response to standing
- Diastolic blood pressure response to sustained handgrip

Other cardiovascular tests
- 24 hour heart rate variation
- Power spectral analysis
- Spontaneous baroreflex sensitivity
- Cardiac radionuclide imaging

pressure in response to a range of physiological stimuli that reflect changes in parasympathetic and sympathetic outflow to the heart and blood vessels. They can be performed in the consulting room or at the bedside using a blood pressure device and an ECG machine to record the R-R interval. Previously it was felt that the heart rate tests assessed parasympathetic function and blood pressure test sympathetic function, and that parasympathetic abnormalities preceded abnormalities of sympathetic function, but using more sophisticated tests it is clear that many of these tests asses both branches of the autonomic nervous system and that damage to the sympathetic activity occurs in parallel to parasympathetic damage.

11.3.1 **Heart rate response to deep breathing**

The heart rate response to deep breathing mostly assesses parasympathetic function. Several different techniques of deep breathing are described, but paced deep breathing, e.g. at six breaths per minute, is probably most reliable. Similarly, several different measures of heart rate variation during deep breathing have been described.

11.3.2 **Heart rate response to standing**

On initial standing withdrawal of parasympathetic tone increases the heart rate. In response to subsequent blood pressure changes a baroreflex mediated reflex activates sympathetic nerves. In normal subjects there is a rapid increase in heart rate on standing maximal at around the 15th beat with a relative slowing that is maximal around the 30th beat. The ratio of the 30:15th beat should normally be >1.0. In the presence of autonomic neuropathy the increase in heart rate is slower, and the ratio will be <1.0. Refinements of the test include taking measures from 20–40 beats and 5–25 beats, and measuring the ratio of the longest to shortest R-R interval.

11.3.3 **Heart rate response to the Valsalva manoeuvre**

The heart rate response to the Valsalva manoeuvre is influenced by both parasympathetic and sympathetic activity. In normal subjects the response during the strain is vasoconstriction and an increase in heart rate, and there is an overshoot of blood pressure and a slowing of the heart rate following the release of the strain. The patient forcibly exhales against a fixed resistance for 15 seconds and the Valsalva ratio is the ratio of the longest R-R interval after the manoeuvre to the shortest R-R interval during the manoeuvre. In autonomic neuropathy the increase in heart rate during the strain is reduced, so the ratio is reduced.

11.3.4 **Systolic blood pressure response to standing**

A change from lying to standing activates afferent receptors from baroreceptors which increases efferent sympathetic impulses and causes an increase in peripheral vascular resistance and an increase in heart rate, with little change in blood pressure. In patients with autonomic neuropathy baroreflex compensation is impaired so blood pressure falls. A fall in systolic blood pressure of >30 mmHg is abnormal.

11.3.5 **Diastolic blood pressure response to sustained handgrip**

Sustained isometric contraction is tested using a handgrip dynom-eter which asses a reflex arc involving both afferent and efferent fibres from muscles. The efferent fibres innervate the heart and muscle, increasing heart rate, blood pressure and cardiac output. A normal response is an increase in diastolic blood pressure of >15 mmHg, and a rise of <10 mmHg is abnormal.

11.3.6 **Other tests of cardiac function**

There are several other newer tests of the heart that require more sophisticated equipment (Box 11.2). A reduction in 24 hour heart rate variability is thought to be more sensitive than the standard reflex tests and may be able to detect cardiac autonomic neuropa-thy earlier. The sympathetic innervation of the heart can be visual-ized and quantified using the myocardial uptake of the radionuclide meta-iodobenzylguanidine (MIBG), and in cardiovascular autonomic neuropathy there is a decrease in uptake.

11.4 **Prognosis of diabetic autonomic neuropathy**

In patients with diabetic cardiovascular autonomic neuropathy there is an increase in total mortality and sudden death, and in patients with symptomatic autonomic neuropathy mortality may be over 50% on five to ten year follow up. A meta-analysis has shown a greater risk for studies that defined neuropathy with the presence of two or more abnormalities compared with studies that used one measure (Figure 11.2).

Cardio-respiratory arrest is well described in patients with symp-tomatic diabetic autonomic neuropathy, and there are several other possible explanations for the increased mortality associated with diabetic autonomic neuropathy (Box 11.3).

11.4.1 **QT interval prolongation**

Many studies have shown increases in the QT interval in patients with diabetic autonomic neuropathy. In non-diabetic subjects increases in the QT interval are associated with an increased risk of sudden death, so this is one possible linking factor between diabetic autonomic neuropathy and sudden death.

Figure 11.2 Relative risks for studies of cardiovascular autonomic neuropathy (CAN) and mortality

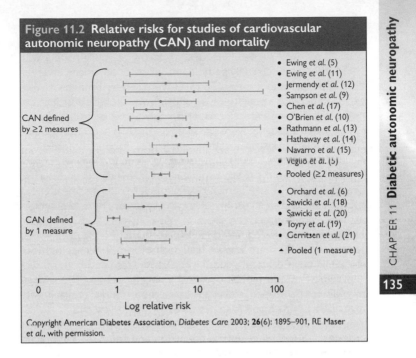

CAN defined by ≥2 measures
- Ewing et al. (5)
- Ewing et al. (11)
- Jermendy et al. (12)
- Sampson et al. (9)
- Chen et al. (17)
- O'Brien et al. (10)
- Rathmann et al. (13)
- Hathaway et al. (14)
- Navarro et al. (15)
- Veglio et al. (5)
- ▲ Pooled (≥2 measures)

CAN defined by 1 measure
- Orchard et al. (6)
- Sawicki et al. (18)
- Sawicki et al. (20)
- Toyry et al. (19)
- Gerritsen et al. (21)
- ▲ Pooled (1 measure)

Log relative risk

11.5 Sudden death in diabetes

Sudden and unexpected death of a young person is a rare but well described occurrence in non-diabetic subjects. It was suggested that the frequency of sudden death in type 1 diabetes increased following the introduction of the use of human insulin into clinical practice, and that this increase was caused by hypoglycaemia. This was subsequently named the 'dead in bed syndrome'. Estimates of sudden death in type 1 diabetes suggest that the risk is double that of the non-diabetic population, but a clear link with hypoglycaemia has not yet been established.

Box 11.3 Possible causes of death in autonomic neuropathy

- concomitant cardiac or renal disease
- absent or altered perception of myocardial ischaemia
- deficient response to stress such as surgery, infection or anaesthesia
- increased predisposition to arrhythmia because of QT interval prolongation
- changes in cardiac sympathetic/parasympathetic balance

11.5.1 'Dead in bed' syndrome

The British Diabetic association, (now Diabetes UK) collected a detailed series of sudden, unexpected deaths of young people with type 1 diabetes, referred by pathologists, diabetes physicians, and relatives of people with diabetes. 53 cases were referred and many were excluded because a definite cause of death was identified such as suicide, self-poisoning, ketoacidosis, or hypoglycaemic brain damage.

Twenty-two patients were classified as 'dead in bed'. They tended to be on multiple insulin injections and free of diabetic complications. All died outside hospital, 19 were sleeping alone at the time of death and 15 died during the night. 20 patients were found in an undisturbed bed. Few had any of the known risk factors for confirmed death from hypoglycaemia (Box 11.4). 14 patients had a history of severe nocturnal hypoglycaemia, and the scenario was consistent with an episode of severe or protracted nocturnal hypoglycaemia having precipitated sudden death. As there was no neuropathological evidence of hypoglycaemic brain damage a sudden cardiac or respiratory arrest was implicated. Post-mortem biochemical testing for possible hypoglycaemia was not performed, and in any case is notoriously unreliable with many false positives and false negatives for hypoglycaemia.

Sudden, unexpected death in patients with type 1 diabetes has now been described in several countries, and some risk factors are suggested (Box 11.4).

11.5.2 **Possible mechanisms of sudden death**

In the general population the most frequent cause of sudden death is a cardiac arrhythmia, mostly related to coronary heart disease.

Box 11.4 Risk factors for death from hypoglycaemia and 'dead in bed' syndrome in type 1 diabetes

Risk factors for death from hypoglycaemia

- alcoholism and/or inebriation
- psychiatric illness or personality disorder
- self neglect or malnutrition
- fecklessness/resistance to education
- diabetes secondary to pancreatic disease
- hypopituitarism following pituitary ablation

Risk factors for 'dead in bed' syndrome

- previous nocturnal hypoglycaemia
- living/sleeping alone
- intensive insulin therapy
- multiple injections of insulin
- alcohol ingestion

> **Box 11.5 Possible mechanisms of sudden death in type 1 diabetes**
>
> **Autonomic neuropathy**
>
> - Prolongation of the QT interval
> - Reduced heart rate variability
> - Diminished baroceptor sensitivity.
>
> **Hypoglycaemia**
>
> - Activation of the autonomic nervous system
> - Increased plasma epinephrine and lowering of serum potassium
> - Prolongation of the QT interval
> - Autonomic imbalance during hypoglycaemia.

Some of the increase in sudden death in diabetes will be the consequence of premature coronary heart disease, but this was excluded in the cases described. In some patients hypoglycaemic convulsions may contribute, but again this was circumstantially excluded by the fact that most subjects were found in an undisturbed bed.

The two additional possible contributions to sudden death in diabetes are autonomic neuropathy and hypoglycaemia. A plausible explanation is a combination of the changes in the QT interval which accompany nocturnal hypoglycaemia but fails to waken the patients unless symptoms are intense, occurring on a background of early autonomic neuropathy, provoking fatal arrhythmia (Box 11.5).

11.6 Treatment of diabetic autonomic neuropathy

Intensive glycaemia control can slow the development and progression of autonomic neuropathy in type 1 and type 2 diabetes. Some drugs have been shown to improve measures of autonomic dysfunction, including the beta-blocker metoprolol, the ACE inhibitor quinapril, and the angiotensin-II receptor antagonist losartan, but the long term effects on mortality are not known.

There is a strong association between autonomic neuropathy and microalbuminuria, and there has recently been suggested a paradigm for treating diabetic patients with autonomic dysfunction (Figure 11.3). Before this is accepted into routine practice, however, studies are required to see if these pharmacological interventions consistently improve autonomic function, and whether this translates into better exercise tolerance or reduced mortality, and this approach should be considered experimental at present.

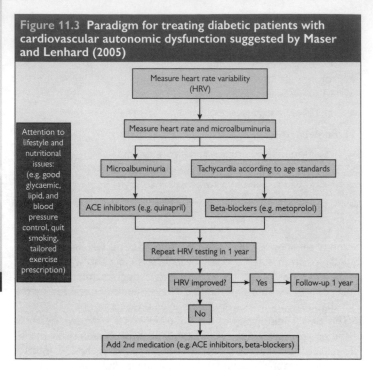

Figure 11.3 Paradigm for treating diabetic patients with cardiovascular autonomic dysfunction suggested by Maser and Lenhard (2005)

11.7 Conclusions

Abnormalities of cardiovascular autonomic neuropathy are common on testing of cardiovascular reflexes, but symptomatic autonomic neuropathy is uncommon, and carries a poor prognosis. Large multicentre studies are required of possible pharmacological interventions to reduce the high cardiovascular mortality associated with symptomatic autonomic neuropathy.

References

Fisher M, Heller SR (2007) Mortality, cardiovascular morbidity and possible effects of hypoglycaemia on diabetic complications. In: BM Frier and M Fisher, eds. *Hypoglycaemia in Clinical Diabetes*, pp. 265-83, John Wiley & Sons, Ltd, Chichester, UK.

Maser RE, Lenhard MJ (2005) Cardiovascular autonomic neuropathy due to diabetes mellitus: clinical manifestations, consequences, and treatment. *Journal of Clinical Endocrinology and Metabolism* **90**: 5896–903.

Maser RE, Mitchell BD, Vinik AI, Freeman R (2003) Cardiac autonomic neuropathy in diabetes. A clinical perspective. *Diabetes Care* **26**: 1895–901.

Pop-Busui R (2010) Cardiac autonomic neuropathy in diabetes. A clinical perspective. *Diabetes Care* **33**: 434–41.

Tatersall RB, Gill GV (1991) Unexplained deaths of type 1 diabetic patients. *Diabetic Medicine* **8**: 49–58.

Vinik AI, Maser RE, Mitchell BD, Freeman R (2003) Diabetic autonomic neuropathy. *Diabetes Care* **26**: 1553–79.

Vinik AI, Ziegler D (2007) Diabetic cardiovascular autonomic neuropathy. *Circulation* **115**: 387–97.

Chapter 12

Health economic aspects of treating cardiovascular disease in diabetes

Ailsa Brown, Joyce Craig, and Ken Paterson

> ### Key points
>
> - Scarce resources in health care systems mean that choices have to be made on how resources are spent
> - Economic evaluations are increasingly used in health-care decision making to provide an indication of the cost-effectiveness of different treatment options
> - The cost-effectiveness ratios of treatments for glycaemic control, lipid-lowering, blood pressure control and management of established cardiovascular disease are generally within a range that is considered cost-effective in the UK.

12.1 Economic evaluation of health care

Health economic assessments are increasingly being used in health care decision-making, as evidenced by the use of economic analyses by organisations such as the National Institute for Health and Clinical Excellence (NICE) and the Scottish Medicines Consortium (SMC). Their use relates to a basic problem in economics, resolving the issues of scarcity and choice. Scarcity of resources exists in health care systems worldwide and means that there will never be sufficient funds to meet all the competing demands for health care. Choices therefore have to be made about how to spend resources in order to meet the objectives of the health care system. Economic evaluation techniques can provide a systematic way of considering solutions to the problem of scarcity and choice by allowing comparison of the costs and consequences of two (or more) alternative health care interventions.

12.1.1 **The incremental cost-effectiveness ratio (ICER)**

It is clear from the preceding chapters that there are many different treatments available to treat cardiovascular disease in people with diabetes; each treatment will give rise to a specific pattern of costs and effects. For example, in trying to manage a patient's weight, clinicians could use lifestyle interventions or drug therapy. If drug therapy provided greater benefits but at an increased cost compared to lifestyle modification, then economic evaluation can provide a marker to help the decision-maker judge whether the additional benefits justify the additional costs. In comparing treatment options in an economic evaluation, the convention is to calculate the additional benefit provided by the more effective treatment and then present the findings in terms of 'cost per additional unit of benefit' e.g. 'cost per additional life year gained'. This ratio of incremental cost to incremental benefit is known as the incremental cost-effectiveness ratio (ICER).

12.1.2 **Quality Adjusted Life Year (QALY)**

Many treatments offer a range of effects such as improved quality of life and prolonged survival. Cost-effectiveness analysis using an outcome measure such as a 'cost per additional life year gained' struggles to take account of both dimensions of benefit. Another commonly used measure of benefit seen in economic evaluations is the quality adjusted life year (QALY). The QALY adjusts length of life for quality of life by assigning a value between zero and one (where zero represents death and one represents perfect health) for each year of life. Figure 12.1 illustrates the concept of a QALY.

Without the new health technology the individual's quality of life, measured on the y axis, would deteriorate over time until they

Figure 12.1 **Diagram of the concept of QALY (quality-adjusted life years)**

die ('death 1'). However, with the technology the individual's quality of life is maintained at a higher level and they survive some years longer than with the original treatment ('death 2'). Area A represents the quality of life gain with the new treatment while area B corresponds to the survival gain with the treatment. Added together, they represent the total QALY gain associated with the new treatment. QALYs thus have the advantage of capturing gains in quality of life and survival in a single measure.

12.1.3 Health economic models

Data from a variety of sources (clinical trials, disease registries, epidemiological studies) are often combined to develop a health economic model of the disease and the effects of interventions. Costs of the new treatment can be offset by savings from adverse events avoided as well as the clinical benefits of improved quality of life and survival. Benefits are often extrapolated beyond the data that are available (e.g. from a 2-year clinical trial to 10 years or even patient lifetime) and this, along with other aspects of the modelling, requires assumptions to be made. The impact of varying these assumptions, either individually or in combination, is tested in sensitivity analyses, giving a range of ICERs from best to worst case scenarios. This reveals which assumptions are key to the cost per QALY and may allow key assumptions to be underpinned by additional data.

To assess if the treatment is cost-effective, the resulting 'cost per QALY' ratio can be compared either to similar ratios for other interventions already adopted by the health service or to the decision-maker's stated willingness to pay for an additional QALY. In the UK, NICE uses a rule of thumb that a cost per QALY of less than £20,000 is generally considered to be cost-effective.

The remainder of this chapter will discuss the findings of selected published economic evaluations on the principal treatment options in this population.

12.2 Cost-effectiveness of improved glycaemic control

12.2.1 Glycaemic control in type 1 diabetes

The Diabetes Control and Complications Trial (DCCT) is discussed in Chapter 2. Alongside this clinical trial, an economic evaluation was conducted. An economic model was developed to estimate the lifetime benefits and costs of intensive insulin therapy compared to conventional therapy. Data from other clinical trials and epidemiological studies were used to model the probabilities of longer-term complications such as blindness, end-stage renal disease (ESRD) and amputations. The model was structured around the occurrence of events such as retinopathy, nephropathy, neuropathy and death. Intensive insulin therapy was more expensive than conventional care but resulted in fewer deaths and fewer expensive-to-treat micro-vascular complications. The resulting cost per QALY gained was $19,987 (at 1994 US dollars), leading the authors to conclude that intensive insulin therapy is a cost-effective treatment option.

12.2.2 Glycaemic control in type 2 diabetes

UKPDS has also been discussed in Chapter 2. An economic evalu-ation was an integral part of this trial. As with DCCT, information from the trial was combined with other data to estimate the lifetime costs and effects of the various treatment options considered in the trial. Microvascular and macrovascular complications were included in the model. The cost per QALY gained from intensive treatment compared to conventional treatment was £6,028. The use of met-formin in overweight patients was found to be both cheaper and more effective than conventional treatment. These results suggest that the intensive blood glucose control strategies studied in UKPDS should be considered cost-effective compared to other accepted uses of health care funds in the UK. The results rely on the results of UKPDS and it should be noted that, as UKPDS was conducted between 1977 and 1991, standards of conventional care are likely have improved. This may affect the relative costs and effects of inten-sified glycaemic control compared to current conventional care.

12.2.3 Cost effectiveness of other anti-diabetic drugs in type 2 diabetes

Several economic evaluations have investigated the cost-effective-ness of adding a thiazolidinedione to existing treatments. A study based on the PROactive trial estimated that the cost per QALY gained from adding pioglitazone to existing treatment in patients at a high risk of cardiovascular events was £4,060. This analysis was based on the Centre for Outcomes Research (CORE) diabetes model, which has been used in several economic evaluations in diabetes. In the model, any improvement in baseline HbA_{1c} as a result of a novel treatment is assumed to be sustained. There is the possibility that, while an improvement in HbA_{1c} may be observed over the short-to-medium term, this improvement may be eroded in the longer term, which could alter (increase) the stated ICER.

The model also assumes that the benefits of lowered HbA_{1c} are the same irrespective of which treatment has led to the lowering. Recent controversy around data on rosiglitazone has cast doubt on this assumption, and while similar doubts have not been raised for other oral agents it is a useful reminder that health economic assess-ments depend on the validity of the clinical inputs to the analysis.

The cost-effectiveness of adding sitagliptin or a sulphonylurea to metformin was compared in patients with poorly controlled HbA_{1c}

across six European countries. The clinical data for the sulphonylurea comparisons came from an unpublished per protocol analysis of a clinical study. The analyses used the UKPDS model. Sitagliptin was reported to be cost-effective compared with adding a sulphonylurea with incremental cost per QALYs ranging from €5,949 to €20,350 across the countries.

12.2.4 Cost-effectiveness of the self monitoring of blood glucose in type 2 diabetes

Data from the randomized controlled trial (RCT) diabetes glycaemic education and monitoring (DiGEM), set in the UK, reported that additional self monitoring of blood glucose alone, or with training in self interpretation of the results, compared to standard care, was associated with similar clinical outcomes, higher costs and lower quality of life in patients with non-insulin treated type 2 diabetes. The study concluded self monitoring of blood glucose, in addition to usual care, was unlikely to be cost-effective This result provides the NHS with the opportunity to disinvest from this activity and use the money more effectively.

12.3 Cost-effectiveness of blood pressure control in type 2 diabetes

In addition to investigating the cost-effectiveness of glycaemic interventions, tight blood pressure control was also investigated as part of UKPDS. A policy of tight blood pressure control was associated with a cost per QALY gained of £369 compared to a less tight blood pressure control target, reflecting the low costs of the drugs used in blood pressure management in UKPDS. This very low ICER would not apply to use of newer, more expensive blood pressure lowering drugs which may, however, also offer additional benefits over the drugs used in UKPDS.

12.4 Cost-effectiveness of statin therapy for primary and secondary prevention of CVD in people with diabetes

A recent health technology assessment compared statin therapy to no treatment for people with diabetes. The analysis assumed statins achieved a similar relative risk reduction from baseline CVD event rates for people with diabetes and those without diabetes. Because people with diabetes are at higher absolute risk of CVD events the absolute benefit, measured by events avoided, is greater for this group.

For those with diabetes and a history of CVD, the incremental cost per QALY was below £9,000 for all age groups. For primary CVD prevention in people with diabetes, the incremental cost per QALY was under £17,500 for all aged less than 75 years old, rising to £27,600 for men aged 85 years.

The analysis used a weighted average annual cost of statins of £317. Simvastatin has since become available as a generic product and its annual cost has fallen from the £297 used in the model to under £50. The sensitivity analyses in the assessment showed that a 40% reduction in price was associated with a 36% reduction in the cost per QALY. The cost per QALY with generic simvastatin will be even lower than this as the ICER is clearly very sensitive to drug cost. These analyses suggest that treatment with statins is cost-effective for primary and secondary prevention of CVD in all people with diabetes.

This conclusion is supported by a more recent analysis of the cost-effectiveness of giving 40 mg simvastatin daily to almost 6,000 people with diabetes, 90% of whom had type 2 diabetes. These were included in a randomized controlled trial of 20,536 people. The economic evaluation combined the clinical trial data and UK hospital admission event costs, using an annual cost for simvastatin of £63.50. The results showed that lifetime use of the statin was cost-saving for people with type 2 diabetes (i.e. the cost of the sim-vastatin was less than the savings from the hospitalization events avoided).

146

12.5 **Cost-effective strategies to manage people with diabetes and established CVD**

Established CVD includes patients with ST-segment elevation myocardial infarction and non-ST-segment elevation acute coronary syndromes (ACS). The main management strategies are medical therapy or early primary angioplasty. Choices within the latter include primary angioplasty with bare metal stents or drug-eluting stents, or coronary artery bypass surgery. This section reviews the evidence on the cost-effectiveness of these strategies.

12.5.1 **Cost-effective management of people with diabetes and ST-segment elevation myocardial infarction**

Data from a UK observational database (n = 3,002 patients, of whom 440 (15%) had diabetes) estimated the cost-effectiveness of primary angioplasty compared with thrombolysis for ST elevation myocardial infarction. The treatment costs and delays to treatment observed were incorporated into a model that synthesized evidence from 22 RCTs. Angioplasty-based care had an incremental cost of

£4,520 per QALY gained and a 90% probability of being cost-effective at a threshold of £20,000 per QALY gained. This confirmed the findings of earlier studies.

12.5.2 Cost-effective management of people with diabetes and non ST- segment elevation ACS

An economic evaluation assessed the cost-effectiveness of routine angiography, followed by revascularization if clinically indicated and a conservative strategy, across risk group. The model was based on RCT data. Patients with diabetes were classified as high risk. For this group, the early interventional strategy had a 95% probability of being cost-effective at a threshold of £20 000 per QALY.

12.6 Cost-effectiveness of surgical interventions for weight loss in overweight people with type 2 diabetes

Clinical studies suggest that bariatric surgery in obese patients with type 2 diabetes can, in some cases, result in complete resolution of diabetes. A recent health technology appraisal carried out an economic analysis of bariatric surgery compared to non-surgical management of moderate to severe obesity in patients with type 2 diabetes. The results indicated that bariatric surgery would generally be considered cost-effective. If the benefits of treatment were considered short-term (2 years) the cost per QALY was £18,930, falling to £1367 if the benefits were considered to arise over a 20 year time horizon.

147

12.7 Conclusions

This brief review of the cost-effectiveness of selected treatments for people with diabetes supports prescribing statins for primary prevention and angioplasty rather than medical management for initial treatment of acute coronary syndromes. Strategies of intensive blood glucose control and tight blood pressure control are also cost-effective uses of health care resources. New interventions will have to demonstrate clinical benefits to justify any increased cost relative to existing proven managements.

References

Bravo Vergel Y, Palmer S, Asseburg C, et al. (2007) Is primary angioplasty cost effective in the UK? Results of a comprehensive decision analysis. *Heart* **93**: 1238–43.

Clarke PM, Gray AM, Briggs A, Stevens RJ, Matthews DR, Holman RR on behalf of the UK Prospective Diabetes Study (2005) Cost-utility analysis of intensive blood glucose and tight blood pressure control in type 2 diabetes (UKPDS 72). *Diabetologia* **48**: 868–77.

Diabetes Control and Complications Trial Research Group (1996) Lifetime benefits and costs of intensive therapy as practiced in the diabetes control and complications trial. *Journal of the American Medical Association* **276**: 1409–15.

Drummond MF, Sculpher MJ, Torrance GW, O'Brien BJ, Stoddart GL (2005) *Methods for the Economic Evaluation of Health Care Programmes* 3rd edn, Oxford University Press, Oxford.

Heart Protection Study Collaborative Group (2006) Lifetime cost effectiveness of simvastatin in a range of risk groups and age groups derived from a randomised trial of 20 536 people. *British Medical Journal* **333**: 1145(2 December), doi:10.1136/bmj.38993.731725.BE (published 10 November 2006).

Hill R, Bagust A, Bakhai A, et al. (2004) Coronary artery stents: a rapid systematic review and economic evaluation. *Health Technology Assessment* **8**(35): 1–242.

Henriksson M, Epstein DM, Palmer SJ et al. (2008) The cost-effectiveness of an early interventional strategy in non-ST-elevation acute coronary syndrome based on the RITA 3 trial. *Heart* **94**: 717–23.

Picot J, Jones J, Colquitt JL, et al. (2009) The clinical effectiveness and cost-effectiveness of bariatric (weight loss) surgery for obesity: a systematic review and economic evaluation. *Health Technology Assessment* **13**(41): 1–190.

Robinson M, Palmer S, Sculpher M, et al. (2005) Cost-effectiveness of alternative strategies for the initial medical management of non-ST elevation acute coronary syndrome: systematic review and decision-analytical modeling. *Health Technology Assessment* **9**(27): 1–158.

Sculpher MJ, Petticrew M, Kelland KL, Elliott RA, Holdright DR, Buxton MJ (1998) Resource allocation for chronic stable angina: a systematic review of effectiveness, costs and cost-effectiveness of alternative interventions. *Health Technology Assessment* **2**(10): 1–176.

Simon J, Gray A, Clarke P, Wade A, Neil A, Farmer A on behalf of the Diabetes Glycaemic Education and Monitoring Trial Group (2008) Cost effectiveness of self monitoring of blood glucose in patients with non-insulin treated type 2 diabetes: economic evaluation of data from the DiGEM trial. *British Medical Journal* **336**: 1177, 10.1136/bmj.39526.674873. BE (published 17 April 2008).

Valentine WJ, Bottomley JM, Palmer AJ, et al. on behalf of the PROactive Study Group (2007) PROactive 06: cost-effectiveness of pioglitazone in type 2 diabetes in the UK. *Diabetic Medicine* **24**: 982–1002.

Wailoo A, Goodacre S, Sampson F et al. (2010) Primary angioplasty versus thrombolysis for acute ST-elevation myocardial infarction: an economic analysis of the National Infarct Angioplasty Project. *Heart* **96**: 668–72.

Ward S, Lloyd Jones M, Pandor A, et al. (2007) A systematic review and economic evaluation of statins for the prevention of coronary events. *Health Technology Assessment* **11**(14): 1–160.

Index

151